THANKSGIVING

THANKSGIVING

AN AIDS
JOURNAL

ELIZABETH COX

1817

HARPER & ROW, PUBLISHERS, New York
Grand Rapids, Philadelphia, St. Louis, San Francisco
London, Singapore, Sydney, Tokyo, Toronto

Designer: Cassandra J. Pappas

Library of Congress Cataloging-in-Publication Data

Cox, Elizabeth, 1953–

Thanksgiving : an AIDS journal / by Elizabeth Cox.
    p.   cm.
ISBN 0-06-016230-9
1. Avedon, Keith—Health.   2. Cox, Elizabeth, 1953–   .   3. AIDS (Disease)—Patients—United States—Biography.   4. AIDS (Disease)—Patients—United States—Family relationships.   5. Wives—United States—Biography.   I. Title.
RC607.A26A943   1990
362.1'969792'0092—dc20

[B]   89-33764

---

90 91 92 93 94 VB/HD 10 9 8 7 6 5 4 3 2

This book is dedicated
to the memory of my husband,
KEITH DUGGAN AVEDON,
1947–1987

THANKSGIVING

There is no space in this apartment. It is so claustrophobic in these two rooms that this evening I find myself thinking fondly of Keith's room in Intensive Care. That's really crazy. I am thinking of his room at night. I remember it as open and large, even though it was a glassed-in cubicle. It was silent and desolate in there. Just the hiss and click of the respirator. And the sound of my own prayers in my head.

I remember sitting by Keith's bed, touching him, and thinking, "I have to tell Keith about this. I can't wait to tell Keith about this." Then I would remember that I was holding his hand, that he was there with me. But he wasn't really there. I would get chills, shiver, shake myself as if I were trying to wake myself up from a bad dream. But it wasn't a dream. I couldn't wake up or move away. Each day I had to keep putting one leaden foot in front of the other and go on.

People have said to me that they think Keith pulled through because of the things I said to him then. I remember trying to think of things to say that would make him want to live. But I don't remember saying them. I remember feeling that I had to feed Keith—nourish him—with the sound of my voice. But I don't remember hearing myself speak. It was as if my words were sucked into a vacuum. When I think of that room I think of silence.

I remember standing outside his door before entering. Having finished putting on my gown and gloves, I would pause for a moment and take a deep breath—feeling as if the breath I took had to last me until I came out of the room again. I was going where there was no oxygen. I had to take it with me.

But holding Keith's hand felt good. It always felt good. Even when his feet were wrapped in foil and the windows were wide open and his eyes had floated up into his head, his hand felt good. It felt like Keith.

I don't understand how all this happened. I remember waking up in the middle of the night at Montauk. Last August. Three months before Keith collapsed in London. We were on vacation. We were really enjoying ourselves. But the last few nights at the beach I would wake up in the middle of the night and a voice would say to me, "Keith is dying." Then I'd put my head on his shoulder and smell his skin. I thought his sweat smelled funny, but if I really thought about it I couldn't smell anything at all. I'd start sobbing. I'd get up and splash cold water on my face and tell myself I must be losing my mind. This must be delayed post-partum depression. Look in the bedroom. There's Luke. There's Keith. Everyone is fine.

4

Our last afternoon in Montauk while Luke was napping Keith and I were making love and I found a shingles blister on Keith's back.

Then we came home from Montauk and things got really crazy. Keith started getting fevers at night sometime in September. He had had polio when he was a very young child. We both became afraid that he had post-polio syndrome because he didn't seem to have the same stamina, the same energy, that he usually had. Keith couldn't relax; he was obsessing about the Chanel job. He was being evasive, doctors were being evasive. Something seemed very, very wrong.

Something was wrong. Why didn't I see it? We could have been closer, together. I remember arguing about things that should have been discussed. I remember walking with Keith, on our way back from taking Luke to the playground, and saying that I wanted to move our bed into the living room, that I missed our pre-baby sex life. I had been feeling that Keith was distracted, that since our return from Montauk Keith had seemed ambivalent about our sex life. I thought that moving our bed out of the bedroom, away from Luke's crib, would help. Keith said it didn't matter. He said I was making an issue out of nothing. That made me angry. We argued. Keith seemed far away. Preoccupied.

We celebrated our eleventh wedding anniversary soon after we got home from Montauk. We went out to dinner. Keith wasn't himself. And he wasn't just not feeling well; there was an aura about him. An aura of anxiety so intense that we didn't talk about it. As if out of some unconscious respect for it—or fear of it—we couldn't mention it.

On our wedding anniversaries we always used to tell each other stories—about how crazy life is. Keith would say, "When I write the book about my life . . ." But this anniversary something peculiar was going on; we never relaxed and took stock the way we used to. That night we talked about Luke. Keith talked about his Chanel job (a musical arrangement for a Chanel television commercial which was to be recorded in Europe). He said he was worried about it. We talked about other things too that night, but not about what was really on our minds. Or, in my case, what was below the surface, not having come into consciousness yet. Both of us were ready to go home before the hour we'd told the babysitter we'd be back, which was very unlike us. And when we got home we didn't try to be alone. We took off our shoes, said good-bye to the sitter, and stood over Luke's crib. We watched him sleep.

Keith had had his shingles treated by a dermatologist, who said that he should have a physical because shingles were unusual in a young man. Soon after seeing the dermatologist Keith started feeling achy and having occasional fevers. He also developed a persistent cough. He then went to his regular doctor, who said he had a bronchial infection, for which he prescribed an antibiotic. But, when Keith started taking the antibiotic, his fever went up and he developed a rash. It turned out that the antibiotic had penicillin in it, even though it was written in his file that he was allergic to penicillin. We thought that explained everything. Furious at his doctor, Keith went to a new, highly recommended doctor, Dr. Cohen, who did lots of tests, said he had hepatitis, and gave him the O.K. to leave for Europe.

The afternoon Dr. Cohen told Keith he had hepatitis he arrived home from his appointment a couple of hours later than I had expected him. After he told me the diagnosis, I asked him why he was so late. He said that he had stopped in a church on the way home. The child of a Jewish father and Catholic mother, Keith had been raised Catholic. Although we went to church together at Christmas and Easter, neither of us went regularly. Nevertheless, religion is a very private and strong underpinning in Keith's life. It fulfills a need in him to step away from and evaluate the events in his life, to give thanks or pray. He occasionally went to church when I was pregnant; he sometimes went when he was in the midst of a composing project.

But his going to church that particular afternoon didn't make sense to me. Serious as hepatitis is, it isn't terminal. Did he go to church because he was relieved? Was he going to church because he was nervous about leaving his wife and baby for a couple of weeks to work in Europe?

It was consistent with the mood of those days that I never asked. Often in the month before he left for Europe I felt as if I were watching Keith rather than communicating with him. Perhaps I didn't want to know why he felt the need to go to church. I told myself that the general uneasiness of those days could be accounted for by the stress inherent in the work he was doing.

The Chanel job (and the trip to Europe it entailed) meant so much to Keith. It symbolized success to him. He was being paid a lot of money for his musical skills. It was an indication that he was going to be able to support a family on his music. That was very important to Keith. He had been afraid that having a baby might be the end of his creativity, our creativity, the music in our home, the music in our lives. It was gratifying to Keith that he was working with his cousin Dick. Dick was the only member of the Avedon family Keith looked up to. He had always admired Dick's ability to lead an artistically true life while being commercially successful. When Keith got the Chanel job he felt that he, too, might be able to do that.

Packing for this trip was like getting ready for the future, a successful future. The only hitch was that he was worried about his health. We both were. But Dr. Cohen had said he had hepatitis, so that seemed to explain all his recent problems. We thought he could get strong after the job was finished.

The night Keith left for Rome I carried Luke downstairs to see the limousine, to say good-bye. While Keith showed the limousine to Luke, I had to run off to the pharmacy to pick up a cough-medicine prescription. I was worried. It struck me that my formerly healthy husband couldn't go off to Europe without a bag of medicines. What was happening to him? What did his persistent cough have to do with hepatitis? How long would the hepatitis last? Why did Keith feel fine one day and have a fever the next?

Luke kissed Keith good-bye and wouldn't let go of his neck. He was really wailing when Keith left. It seemed so wrong, Keith going off in the night.

And I remember Keith calling from Rome and me not wanting to talk to him. I didn't want to know how he was; I didn't want to start worrying again. He said that he was doing O.K. but that the previous evening he had been out and gotten so dizzy he had to take a cab back to the hotel. My legs started to shake. Why did I feel so frightened?

Two nights later Luke woke up in the middle of the night, around 1 A.M. While I was changing his diaper, getting ready to put him back in the crib, the phone rang. The machine was on. Whoever it was hung up. I told myself it was a wrong number, but I couldn't sleep the rest of the night.

At 7 A.M. Keith's hotel in London called to say Keith had been taken to the hospital. I called the hospital, trying to reach Keith. The woman who answered the phone said to call Admitting. I called my mother. I heard my voice shaking. "Keith has been taken to the hospital. Please come over right away, I can't make calls to London with Luke around. He sees how upset I am and it's making him crazy."

She arrived around eight. She played with Luke while I called the hospital. What did it mean, the doctor saying, "Your husband is a very sick man"? I asked if I should leave for London, get to him. "Your husband is a very sick man." Was he in danger? "Your husband is a very sick man." What was wrong? "Your husband is a very sick man." Why weren't they being straight with me? They were keeping something from me, I felt sure.

Then Keith called. He was coughing and gasping for breath. He kept having to put down the phone to pick up an oxygen mask. He said that the doctors didn't know what he had, but they thought it might be Legionnaires disease. They had told him that he would have to be in the hospital for at least three weeks. He sounded confused and scared. It was hard for him to talk. He gave me the name of the doctor in charge of his case. I said I would call him and have Dr. Cohen, his New York doctor, call him too. We hung up.

Talking to Keith was terrifying, especially after the ominous conversation with the doctor, but it was my conversation with the doctor whose name I got from Keith that put the seal on my anxiety, froze the panic in my bones. Like the first doctor, he wouldn't tell me what was wrong. He too just kept saying: "Your husband is very sick." But he went a step further: when I asked him if I should go to Keith he said he thought that was a good idea.

I called Dr. Cohen to ask her to call the English doctors. She was so relentlessly cheerful in the midst of my terror that I felt myself become angrier and angrier until suddenly I heard myself asking her if Keith had AIDS. "Whatever makes you think that?" she chirped in a manner I found condescending and infuriating. I didn't know, but I did know that something was terribly wrong with my husband—something that made Dr. Cohen's response seem empty.

My mother said that she would go with me to London. She,

Luke, and I should just pack up and go. But how did we do it? I don't remember much. Only that a terrible numbness set in, as if I had walked into something like a black steel wall that took away my senses. Mother took Luke to the park so I could make the necessary arrangements—plane reservations, hotel reservations, passports.

Then I was changing Luke's diaper. My mother was standing next to me, and I heard myself once again saying, "What if Keith has AIDS?" My mother said, "Don't be silly, how could Keith have AIDS? Whatever makes you think that?" She was echoing Dr. Cohen. I felt desperate, frustrated, angry. And I meant it when I said, "I don't know, how do I know?" I truly didn't know why I had now said that dread word twice in a matter of hours, but saying it had made it seem real, a real possibility. Too real. So I tried to push it back into the darkness from which it had come, as if not thinking about it could make it go away.

We got on a night flight to Heathrow. When Luke had finally settled down to sleep it occurred to me that there was nothing further I could do now. I was over the ocean. No news could get to me. I could have a drink and try to sleep. But I was scared to go to sleep. Sleeping would mean losing control. And it would make the time pass more quickly when part of me was wishing the plane ride would go on forever.

Westminster Hospital is very old. Wooden floors and creaky wooden stairs. Tall dark ceilings. A door with a bell to ring to get into Intensive Care. A young, pretty nurse. "Please go to the room at the end of the hall. The head sister wants to talk to you." Sister? It took me a minute to recall that all the nurses in England are called sisters. Everything seemed so foreign in that hospital.

"Your husband has very severe pneumonia. We put him on a respirator because he couldn't breathe on his own. When you see him he will not be able to talk to you. I will take you to see him. We are taking all precautions until we know what he has."

Paper gown, paper mask and gloves. Contagion warnings on the door to his cubicle. Where is my Keith?

My panic left when I entered. It was Keith. He was there. I was there with him. I kissed his shoulder, held his hand. His eyes were alert and thankful and relieved I had arrived. I said that everything would be all right. We would pull through. Luke was in London too. Look, here are some pictures of him. I told him that the sister had said that the doctors would know what was wrong with him tomorrow, that I had an appointment to talk to the doctors tomorrow.

Keith had a clipboard, paper, and pen on his stomach. He kept trying to write notes to me, tell me what had happened. I couldn't read his writing—it was too shaky, didn't make sense. It was too hard to try to communicate that way. I held his hand and stroked his forehead. Tried to hold on to the initial feeling of relief I had had when I walked in the door. For at that moment all that had mattered was that I had made it to him, was with him.

But back at the hotel panic hit hard. What was going on? What were the doctors going to say? How could I sleep? There were phone calls to make—Keith's family. I needed someone of Keith's blood here, with me, in the hotel. Keith's sister, Pat, should come. I wanted her with me. She said she would get on the next flight out of New York and arrive the following morning. Get her a room. Get Keith's belongings picked up from his hotel. I must sleep. Must be strong with the doctors tomorrow. Luke. I want to curl up in his crib with him.

The phone rang at around five in the morning. It was Dick,

calling from New York. He said, "You know Keith is going to beat this, don't you, Betsy?" I believed him, fell into a deep, deep sleep.

My mother took Luke to St. James's Park later that morning. I went to the hospital. Keith was completely out of it. I went back to the hotel to collect myself before my meeting with the doctors that afternoon. Pat arrived just in time to leave for the hospital with me. I was glad to see her, but I'm sure I didn't express it. So much was happening so fast there was no time to react. I couldn't allow myself to feel anything yet. It was too important to keep control.

We waited for the doctors in the little room down the hall from the entrance to Intensive Care. It was like a closet, with a small couch and three chairs. Three doctors came in. The head nurse, or sister, sat next to me and held my hand. The oldest doctor, Professor Clark, did the talking. He asked me what Keith's health had been like in the past year. I said that a year and a half ago, a few months after our son was born, Keith had had terrible diarrhea. His doctor had diagnosed it as colitis. We thought it was nerves from having a new baby. A year ago Keith seemed to be tired a lot, but basically O.K. He was under a lot of career pressure at the time, so we figured that accounted for his exhaustion. Last August he had had shingles. Then for most of September he had fevers and a cough. One doctor had said he had a bronchial infection and had treated him for that. Another doctor had said he had hepatitis. Professor Clark said, "That is what we expected." As if I wasn't telling him anything new. As if all the doctors Keith had been to were crazy for not knowing what was really wrong with him. As if this was an expected outcome of the last few months. But what *was* the outcome?

"We believe your husband has AIDS. We did a bronchoscopy to see if he has pneumocystis, an opportunistic infection characteristic of AIDS. We didn't want to tell you until the results of the test came back. That is what he has. We don't expect him to live past the weekend. And if he does you are looking at a very grim future. He may live six months if he recovers from the pneumocystis. I have never heard of anyone with AIDS living more than eleven months."

I believed those doctors. They looked so serious I had to believe them. My husband was in the next room unable to breathe.

Professor Clark said more, much more, but I can't remember any of it. I kept thinking, This can't be happening, this is not real. But the tears on my cheeks felt real. And I remember looking at one of the younger doctors, Dr. Barnes, the one introduced to me as the doctor in charge of Keith while he was in Intensive Care, who seemed as if he were going to cry too. He was staring at me and his eyes were filling up with tears. And the sister next to me was squeezing my hand too hard.

Then there was something about the respirator: that Keith would have to come off it eventually. He couldn't stay on it for more than a few more days. If he stayed on it too long he would pick up another infection from it. They were giving him anti-biotics but couldn't be sure they would work. He could be taken off the respirator as soon as there were signs that the antibiotics were working. They had called other hospitals for advice, a treatment. France. They were using the drug Septra. They were thinking of giving Keith steroids to strengthen his body, give it something to fight with until the crisis was over. The next forty-eight hours were crucial.

I couldn't relate to this information; I couldn't understand. But I pleaded, Please, please make him comfortable. Please don't let him feel any pain.

Dr. Barnes was the man who had put Keith on the respirator.

He said that Keith had wanted it. And he said that Keith would want to know what he had. That he should be told he had AIDS.

I said I would tell him. I want these doctors to go away. I want to be with Keith.

Tying the strings on my gown. Putting on my gloves. This moment must be over. Over quickly. Get it out, say it.

Holding Keith's hand. "You have AIDS." His eyes opened wide and froze with panic. "But you will be O.K. You will do this your own way—with the same inspiration and style that you have done everything in your life. The doctors are good. They are looking into all possible treatments. They have called Paris about a new drug. [When I said that Keith arched his back and pointed to his chest as if to say, "Get it for me."] But you are too sick to take it now; it would hurt you too much now. But they are trying everything. It is going to be O.K." I lost heart halfway through my speech. It wasn't because I didn't believe what I was saying; it was because I could not take in the panic that was in Keith's eyes as I spoke.

And then I did start to not believe my own words. How did I know what the doctors were trying, or if they knew what they were doing? AIDS kills. That's what I kept thinking. And that was really all I knew about AIDS. I didn't know how it killed, how it manifested itself, how it progressed. My knowledge of AIDS was limited to what I had read in the newspaper.

But I stopped thinking. As if I'd left my body. As if my soul and strength were going to leave me and go to Keith. As if I could make each breath happen for him. Just listen to the hiss and click of the respirator, I told myself. And keep touching Keith. Keep talking to him. If I can just keep talking, then even in his near coma Keith will somehow hear me and not float away.

It was all right in that room, holding Keith's hand. I bargained: If I don't leave Keith, Keith won't leave me. It was strangely soothing there, searching my mind for events in our life that were special to him, events I could talk to him about to restore him, pull him back into the world of the living, back to me.

Pat took me to the hotel to eat. My mother opened the hotel-room door with a worried, expectant look on her face. Luke was asleep. I blurted out, "It's AIDS." She was stunned into speechlessness. I started crying. Collapsing. I knew that this scene was too much for my mother—it was too much for me. I tried to pull myself together. Act normal. Wash my face and stop crying. My resolve melted when I passed Luke sleeping in his crib. "My baby isn't going to have a daddy. He is going to grow up without a daddy." Luke, hearing me sobbing, woke up and started crying in confusion and fear. My mother picked him up. I opened the closet door. There were Keith's suitcases and brief-case, which my mother had collected from his hotel. A shopping bag of toys Keith must have bought for Luke: a London bus and a doll. Keith's clothes. The smell of Keith.

I took one of Keith's jackets out of his suitcase and fell into bed with it. I wanted it to comfort me but it hurt to hold it—it couldn't help. More sobbing. Luke upset. I am scaring him. I can't touch my son. I hurt too much to comfort my son. When I looked at him he seemed to have come from far away, from another lifetime. Looking at Luke was painful. I knew I had to get away from him so that he would not feel my pain.

I moved into Pat's room, leaving Luke with my mother.

Early the next morning my mother went back to New York with Luke. She and my father would move into our apartment to take care of him until I could come home. I remember looking out my hotel-room window and seeing Luke in my mother's arms as they got into a taxi to go to the airport, going back home. When would I see him again? Under what circumstances?

Pat and I spent that morning at the hospital. When we got back to the hotel my sister Rachel was waiting for us. I had called her in the middle of the night and pleaded with her to come. I couldn't face not having anyone from my family with me. Mother was leaving, Luke was leaving, Keith was dying. All my feelings were on a very basic, instinctual level. I wanted to have my own flesh and blood with me. I wanted my older sister to take care of me. I must have been glad to see her, but the only thing I remember feeling was that she seemed like something I could hold on to while I was falling apart.

I remember the hotel's doctor coming to see me. Rachel must have called him. Pat and Rachel were telling him that my husband was very ill with pneumonia—that it was a shock, that I was hysterical. He gave me a prescription for sleeping pills.

I remember Pat and Rachel trying to comfort me, trying to get me to calm down. I remember them holding my hands and their faces and voices seeming millions of miles away.

Time turned inside itself. The air was thin. The only time I felt connected to my body was during the morning cab ride to the hospital, when my stomach would churn and I would try not to be sick.

The doctors started giving Keith steroids. Within hours of starting them Keith had become rounder, pumped up, his color better. It was very peculiar—he seemed to glow. I was amazed at his beauty when he was so sick.

One night Pat and I stayed late at the hospital. It was grim at 1 A.M. All the lights were low. Keith's night nurse arrived at midnight, looked at the charts, and said, "Bad blood. Bad blood in America. That's how he got this." I knew he was wrong. That couldn't account for it because Keith hadn't had any blood transfusions. But I kept my thoughts to myself—and pushed them out of my mind. Why think about such things now? At a time like this how dare anyone think about anything except how to get Keith well again?

Dick arrived next. Dick, Pat, and I went into Keith's cubicle. Dick held Keith's hand and said that Keith must not worry about Luke. That he would do everything he could to make sure that Luke and I were taken care of. He told Keith that he loved him.

Since the first phone call from England I had felt as if I had just been stabbed—in shock but not in pain. But watching Dick with Keith was the first time I felt that my wound might bleed. That I might have to feel the hurt. But I also felt that this was a scene I didn't ever want to forget because in some crazy way it was good. I loved Dick then. I loved Keith. I thought of Dick and Keith together, working together—only ten days ago they'd been in Rome filming the Chanel commercial—and it occurred to me that this was a good-bye. Dick was acknowledging that something might be over. That things needed to be said. And he was saying them.

We left Keith's cubicle and went into the little room down the hall. I cried. I remember crying on Dick's shoulder and saying that I was scared to be a widow. I remember stumbling on the *w.* Stuttering. And later feeling so guilty that I had spoken as if Keith were going to die. Guilty that I had spoken out loud an acknowledgment that Keith might die. Guilty that I had even thought it in my own mind. And feeling that I must not let it happen again. That it would be some kind of betrayal of Keith. O.K. for Dick to do it, but not for me.

But I went back and forth about that. I thought about what Keith would want. I told the head sister that if Keith was dying I wanted him to have Catholic last rites. The priest arrived almost immediately. I hadn't expected that. The sisters pulled down the shades on the windows of Keith's cubicle. The priest absolved Keith of his sins. Keith was unconscious, a million miles away.

From the moment the priest arrived until Keith came off the respirator two days later I remember that whenever I was with Keith I had the feeling that I was floating over his room, looking down, watching.

Now and then the sisters opened the window in Keith's cubicle to try to cool him off. It was freezing cold and raining outside. When they weren't trying to cool him off they were trying to keep him warm. (That's what the foil on his feet was for, to reflect his body's heat—I think that's what they told me.) Everything seemed so different from hospitals at home. But I had to assume they knew what they were doing. I let them do their job. My job was to be Keith's lifeline—to keep talking to him, keep touching him—to pull him back to me, pull him away from death.

Once Keith reached out, took my hair, and drew it across his lips. It felt like a communion to me: I felt then that I hadn't lost him, that he was holding on.

One night Pat, Rachel, and I stayed up late talking. We talked about old boyfriends and lovers. I talked about the early days of my relationship with Keith, which reminded Pat and me of the other time we had shared a room, fifteen years ago. I was seventeen. She was twenty-seven, which had seemed so adult to me then. We had shared a room in her family's beach house on Long Island. Keith and I had driven out there in the middle of the night. Keith must have been twenty-three, his first year out of music school. I was still in high school. We had arrived at dawn, and Keith's mother had arranged for me to share a room with Pat. Keith was to sleep in his childhood bedroom down the hall. I remember waiting until I thought Pat was asleep to sneak into Keith's room and hoping she wouldn't wake up when I tiptoed back to my bed hours later.

We laughed at these old memories, and I allowed myself to be soothed by Pat's presence and my sister's. We were women without our men, forgetting ourselves in girl talk. But Rachel's and Pat's husbands were far away. Mine was close. Dying. We couldn't forget ourselves for long. Fortified by our laughter, we had the courage to talk about arrangements for Keith's body if he died. We slept with the lights on.

It was Monday morning early when they decided to take the respirator out. Keith had made it through the weekend. His lungs were clearing. And he could breathe on his own. The doctors and nurses were pleased. But when I looked at Keith I felt as if he had begun a descent into hell. They had stopped the steroids and Keith had shriveled. He was gagging, throwing up over all the tubes, which seemed to be everywhere. The nurses would drain his stomach, pumping out the tube that went down his throat into his stomach.

He was crying for help, for medication. I went out of his room and one sister remarked how wonderful it was that Keith had survived, that he was off the respirator. She said I must be thrilled. I felt anything but thrilled. What kind of body had Keith reentered consciousness into? Shriveled and sick. This was suffering, this was pain. What is it that Keith will have to go through? I asked the head sister if he could have some more pain medication, some sleeping pills. She said the best thing for Keith was to be left alone, to fight it out himself. I should go back to the hotel and get some sleep.

The next few days were grim. I guess we all reentered consciousness: Keith retching and moaning, needing the nurses more than he needed me. I beginning to feel my exhaustion, disorientation. I was determined to be with Keith as much as I could, but those next few days it was determination that kept me at his bedside, not instinct as it had been before.

One afternoon Keith was gagging, a nurse was drawing green liquid out of his stomach, and I was the one who threw up. Pat came in to sit with Keith. I went back to the hotel and got in bed.

I would not let myself think about "What now?" I would not listen to anyone's prognosis. Keith and I would make it through. But what was I supposed to do? What was my role? Keith was suffering, and now the nurses could help him much more than I could. I couldn't bear not having a specific function because it left me with time to think and I couldn't bear to think. There were so many questions that I didn't want to ask.

One night Rachel came into Pat's and my room for room-service dinner. She had been talking to our mother on the phone. She said it was hard talking to New York, that Mother had been hounding her about how Keith got AIDS. That made me angry. It seemed so crazy to me. What were they thinking of? How dare they ask something that I hadn't thought of? What did that matter? Why didn't they just want Keith to be well?

I guess I was becoming defensive, self-righteous. Worn down, tired out.

Friday, five days off the respirator, Keith was moved out of Intensive Care to a small private room downstairs. The sisters lifted him into a wheelchair. He sat sunken into himself, his head nodding on his chest, like an old, old man past death, a skeleton covered with skin—a vision of Keith as he would have been at 110, an ancient Keith, a sight that must be a ghastly vision, an apparition, because my Keith is thirty-eight.

One of the nurses came to me and Pat and said there was a counselor in the hospital, John Lande, who wanted to see Keith, see me, see Pat. I felt I had to protect Keith and screen his company. (One afternoon a Catholic priest had stood by Keith's bed while he was retching and said that Keith must pray to be forgiven of his sins.) I didn't want more people around, more people involved. But Pat said yes, she would like to see him. She looked at me as if I were crazy: "Of course we need him." I said all right.

We went into a room where John had just finished lecturing the nurses on AIDS. There were lists of symptoms on a blackboard—Keith's symptoms, in fact. There on the board was the last year of his medical history. Skin problems, fevers, diarrhea. Cut and dried. This disease was no mystery here. Ambiguous symptoms weren't ambiguous anymore. The pieces of the puzzle fit.

John explained AIDS to me and Pat. He seemed harmless. I said he could talk to Keith if he wanted to—I was going back to the hotel. Pat said she wanted to stay and talk to him.

That night Pat and I were in our hotel room eating and talking and suddenly it became silent. Pat turned to me and said, "I've been strong for you, now you have to be strong for me. I have to tell you that Keith has had a homosexual past."

I heard that. Felt it. As if I had been smacked, slapped across the face. I was furious—furious at the whole situation. I threw the clothes on the bed onto the floor—or was it the clothes in the closet onto the floor? I turned to her and screamed, "Why is your family so crazy? Why is there nothing normal? Why are you all so crazy?"

And then I sat down. I grabbed the bottle of wine, a cigarette. I said, "Tell me. I want to know. Nothing will surprise me. Nothing will ever surprise me or shock me again. Tell me."

She said that Keith had lived with a man when he started college, that the summer six years ago when Keith had visited her in Saratoga he had gone to see the man again.

Pat looked so pained, so upset telling me this. She cried. Then she said that Keith's childhood had been a nightmare. She reminded me that he'd been in and out of the hospital for years because of polio. That he'd lived in the hospital for a year beginning when he was two. That he'd had to wear braces on his legs. She remembered him as a little boy lying on the living-room couch with his fists clenched, not crying, not speaking, rigid with unexpressed emotions. I felt she was trying to make me feel sorry for Keith so I wouldn't hold his past against him. Pat spoke of the nightmare of Keith's childhood as if it were an explanation of his actions. She seemed to want me to see the pain Keith had lived with as an excuse for what had happened since.

I didn't want to hear this. This was crazy. This didn't have anything to do with what was happening now. This should go away. This had no place here. Keith was lying in a hospital bed. The only thing that should matter was getting him out of there and bringing him home. Why talk about these other things? And yet, in a funny way, I wanted Pat to talk. To keep talking. I wanted to hear more about Keith—about my Keith. I should know this.

Keith had told me about the pain in his early life. He had told me about his fears of being abandoned when his parents left after each of their weekly visits to see him in the hospital that had been his home for a year. He had told me about his struggle to walk without braces—the endless series of operations and recuperations. I knew that it would be impossible for anyone to escape the repercussions of a childhood like Keith's. I knew that much of Keith's adult life was a reaction to his past. I knew about Keith crying in my arms at night.

But I also knew about his determination, his absolute determination to make life good—better than good—because the past had been so bad. With determination and courage Keith had created a life he was proud of—become a person he was proud of. He expected a lot of himself, he pushed himself hard, but rarely so hard that he couldn't step back and laugh at himself. Keith enjoyed his life. He had taken the pain and forged it into something beautiful, used it to make of himself a sensitive and compassionate man, richly endowed with pride and a sense of humor. These qualities in Keith were dear to me. I cherished them. They were what made him who he was. I held them in my heart.

But apparently there was more. I wanted to hold on to my own knowledge of Keith's past, my own interpretation. I didn't want to think about what Pat was telling me.

And what Pat had told me wasn't enough—nowhere near enough to explain what was going on now. How could what was going on now be accounted for by any rational explanation? What was rational about any of this? I didn't know what to do with this new knowledge. Was it supposed to explain to me why my husband had AIDS? I couldn't seem to get myself to see the connection between this homosexual episode and the 110-pound man lying in the hospital a few blocks away.

This information made me feel horribly intruded upon. My life with Keith had been invaded. And now Pat was saying to me that John Lande had told her that it was to be expected that I would be angry when she told me. What did I care about John Lande's opinion? Or Pat's for that matter? Stop this intruding on Keith and me.

Most of all I wanted it to be Keith who was telling me what he had done. These were private things—between Keith and me. Nobody else should know anything I didn't about Keith. I could believe what Pat was telling me. But why hadn't Keith told me? I was angry and hurt that he hadn't. That's what hurt. How dare he have secrets from me?

In a funny way the hurt was only on the surface. It was only on the surface because I needed to keep it there for the moment. How could I possibly talk to Keith about any of this while he was so sick? How could I allow myself a reaction without having Keith there to talk it out with? Our life was in stop-time. We didn't even know if Keith would ever leave the hospital and go home again. Until the future was clearer I couldn't let my response out, my anger out, my confusion out, so I refused to feel it.

Or, rather, I refused to feel anything for myself. Instead I tried to turn the part of the tragedy that was mine alone—my feeling of betrayal and pain—into a new source of compassion for Keith. So tragic, I thought. This is so tragic for Keith. He didn't want me to know. He wanted me to know only his best. He must have been ashamed of this. Why hadn't he told me? It was because he was ashamed. And that was what hurt. That was the tragedy. Keith who should be so proud had had to suffer with a sense of shame.

When I saw Keith in the hospital the next day I knew I wouldn't talk to him about it. I couldn't, didn't want to. All I said to him was that Pat had talked to me and that it was all right, that it didn't matter. What mattered was getting well. This new information had no place in there with the chart of his fevers and his weak, skeletal body. I told myself that the relationship between Keith and me transcended the implications of a diagnosis of AIDS. The truth was, of course, that I didn't want to think about it. In my effort to accept AIDS I created a taboo of my husband's past.

But my body started becoming rigid with anger and I hated it, hated feeling that anger in me. Part of the anger was that I felt robbed of being able to just hate the disease. Just hate the disease and hate fate. Everything else should be loving Keith, willing him well and strong, supporting him.

I did things to try to prove to myself, to Keith, that I wasn't angry at him. One night I went out in the rain madly looking for a store that was open to buy Keith some warm pajamas because I had convinced myself that he would freeze to death if he spent another night in flimsy hospital pajamas.

I put the hurt and anger out of my mind. Temporarily. Pat and Rachel left. It was as though the crisis-management team was departing. The nightmare was entering a new phase. I was terrified at the way things kept moving forward. I was nervous about sleeping in a room by myself. Who would take care of me? My brother Robert was coming, but a younger brother didn't seem as comforting as an older sister. Minutes after he arrived, however, I knew how glad I was to have him. He checked into the room across the hall from me, and we talked over dinner about how we must get Keith home, how Keith would get well enough to go home.

I took Keith a Walkman so that he could listen to tapes of his own music and of the Rodrigo guitar concerto. I brought him food. I straightened his room. I lay on the bed beside him. I told him what news I had about Luke when it didn't hurt too much to think about him. We talked hospital gossip. We talked about what Keith could manage to eat and about his fevers, about who had called me at my hotel. In other words, we didn't really talk. We talked about the present, but it was a censored present. The only truly relevant subject we talked about was getting home. Together.

Keith said he wanted to make a book to send to Luke. I bought a blank-paged notebook, crayons, and stickers of circus characters. When I arrived in the morning Keith would be leaning over the book drawing flowers, merry-go-rounds, and pictures of Luke's friends. The book began, "When I was away I got sick so I couldn't come home as fast as I wanted but that will all be over soon." It ended with "Now it's time to say good-

bye. Very soon you and I will roughhouse and like two bugs in
a rug we'll have a big hug and learn about the joy of love.
That's the promise from your Daddy."

The counselor, John Lande, kept appearing. A part of me
wished he would go away, another part of me knew we needed
him—for practical reasons if for nothing else. It was John who
had persuaded the hospital to allow Keith to leave his tiny room
at a time when the hospital had been saying that it was too
dangerous for him to go outside his room because he might pick
up some disease. I suspected they were uncomfortable with the
whole situation, didn't know what to do, and perhaps thought
Keith was dangerous to the other patients in addition to being
in danger from them. It was John who made it clear to the
hospital staff that Keith wasn't going to die of a common cold.
Everyday germs weren't going to kill him. He would die of
something much more serious and bizarre. He needed to walk,
get some strength back, not be treated like a caged animal.
John made it clear that Keith didn't present a health threat to
the other patients.

I knew John was having sessions with Keith, but I didn't
know what they were like. I knew Keith didn't look forward to
seeing him. But Keith always seemed more relaxed after John
left. Or maybe he wasn't more relaxed, just more resigned. I
don't know. I never asked. I didn't want to know. I decided
the sessions, like the subject of how Keith got sick, were a
forbidden subject. I told myself Keith and I shouldn't talk about
anything that would upset him because he was so weak. But it
was myself I didn't want to upset. I desperately wanted to hold
on to what was left of my equilibrium.

John kept saying he wanted to see me. I kept saying I was
fine, that it was Keith who needed him.

Then one afternoon I was lying next to Keith on his bed and
I thought about what it had been like looking at my face in the

bathroom mirror back at the hotel after I'd bathed that morning. My morning shower, washing my hair, had been a focus, an anchor to myself since I had arrived in England. It had always felt surprisingly good, revived me, saved me from my nightmares. But that morning it hadn't worked. I was confused by the face I saw in the mirror—confused because I didn't know it. It was thin and hard. I lay next to Keith and wanted to disappear because suddenly I didn't know anything at all, I didn't know who I was anymore or what was going on. And then I started feeling my anger.

That evening when John came to the hospital I said I wanted to talk to him. He went to the head nurse and got the keys to an empty chemotherapy room. (Keith was on a cancer ward.) Orange vinyl chairs and plastic flowers. "Tell me about your anger, Elizabeth. Hit this chair. Hit it." It seemed an abrupt opener—like something he must have read about in a psychology textbook and decided he'd try out on me—but I obeyed him. I hit that chair. And hit it. And cried. And screamed. "How could he do this? How could he do this to me? To Luke?"

I felt better afterward, but not healed. I felt that I had been doing an exercise, acting out fear and anger. And while I was acting, those feelings had become almost tangible. But there was a funny aftertaste to this exercise. Yes, I felt angry at Keith— but the anger at Keith wasn't the real core of my feelings; it was more a symptom. How do you express your anger when it's directed at the unfairness of life itself? I was turning mine against Keith, the obvious target, but screaming it made me feel like a traitor. Yes, I needed to scream for survival, but I wasn't sure that I believed the words that came out. Although they seemed genuine while I was screaming them, they didn't seem relevant after I had stopped. But they were the only words I had to express something that seemed too big to express, so I just went ahead and screamed that I hated Keith, hoping that if I did that maybe I could dry my eyes and love him more.

Professor Clark was scheduled to visit Keith on Tuesdays. Two Tuesday evenings I pleaded unsuccessfully with him to let Keith go home. Just let him out. We would manage. We could take him home on a stretcher if we had to.

I wasn't really sure why he wouldn't let Keith go. I got a lot of confused messages from that doctor. It made sense to me when he said that Keith wasn't strong enough to leave, but that didn't seem to be the only problem. They were always looking for something more. Doing more tests. Waiting for something else to happen. Wait and see. I got the feeling that they didn't know what to do. Didn't want to discharge him in his present condition yet had nothing to treat him with in the hospital. Professor Clark talked about the CMV level in Keith's blood. It was something they had to watch, he kept saying.

Once I told Professor Clark that I was thinking of going home for a few days. If Keith was stable I wanted to fly to New York and see our baby and then come back. Professor Clark started telling me that that would only confuse Luke, that it would be best if I just stayed. I couldn't tell what he was really saying to me—was it Luke or Keith he was concerned about? But, as with so many other things then, I didn't ask because I was afraid to hear the answer.

Then suddenly, out of the blue, Keith got the O.K. to leave. He could leave in forty-eight hours if his fever stayed down. Robert and I made plane reservations, got service for the handicapped from the airline, and hired a car to take us to the airport. Everyone I called in New York sounded thrilled. Robert was thrilled. Keith was relieved. I felt scared. Really scared. This was going to be hard. This was going to take determination—on Keith's part and mine.

The last evening in England John Lande came to the hospital to have a final session, this time with both me and Keith. I was almost looking forward to that session, thinking we'd get a pat on the back, thinking that we'd celebrate a little, relax for once. That wasn't what happened.

John talked about dying. About living while dying. "Keep flowers around, they'll remind you of life." "Watch your son, he'll show you how to live." And he worked to get us to break down. "What do you want to say to Elizabeth, Keith?"

Keith wanted to say he was sorry. It made him sob. He said that when he came home from being out at night our home was so pure it was like heaven. I had felt like heaven. He shook when he said that. And it broke my heart. He said he hated himself for what he had done.

I told him that I loved him, that it didn't matter. And at that moment I really believed it didn't. What mattered, what hurt, was this emaciated, sobbing man. Even though I didn't understand who this man was, what was going on, or what had happened in the past, this was still Keith. My husband. He was still the man I loved. I wanted to think about that. I didn't see how blaming Keith or concentrating on his death was going to help anything.

Keith and I cried together, and I guess that was a step in the right direction. But it was a bottomless pit of tears and I wanted to stay above it. And it seemed to me that John kept making us drown. "Look at Elizabeth's hair, Keith. Doesn't she have beautiful hair?" More sobs. What was the point of making us cry?

A peculiar kind of inertia overtook me when I was packing up. As though I had taken a drug that I hadn't meant to take, that was making me slow, forgetful, stopping my momentum. A kink in the forward progress. I was fearful. I wanted more time. How could I say good-bye to this place before I had understood what had happened here? It was confusing to me to sort through Keith's bags and take out the clothes he would be wearing on the plane. The same bags I had watched him pack only a month ago in New York. The same bags and clothes I had wept over in a closet only three weeks ago.

I hated being in a foreign country. Nothing felt safe in England. Everything felt strange and dangerous. I was homesick. But I didn't feel ready to leave yet.

One afternoon I had left the hospital to go shopping to buy some more warm clothes—a sweater and a nightgown, things that shouldn't have taken much thought. But everything required thinking about in London: how much things cost in pounds rather than dollars, how to get where I was going, whether to look right or left to see if a car was coming when I crossed the street. I didn't have energy to spare for this kind of thinking. I wanted life to be by rote.

That afternoon I had walked to Oxford Street. It was the week before Thanksgiving. I reached Oxford Street and my heart stopped. Christmas decorations were up. Everything looked so oddly familiar. Suddenly I couldn't remember what year it was, how old I was. But I knew I had been here before. And I couldn't move. A memory hurt.

Fourteen years before, Keith and I had lived together for the first time four blocks away from where I stood staring at those Christmas decorations. I had completely forgotten that. This visit had seemed to take place in a completely different universe. But that other time had happened, too. We had lived near Marble Arch on Seymour Street, on the top floor of a townhouse, in two rooms that were being used for storage by a friend's father. Our rooms looked out over the rooftops of London. We had a bedroom with two single mattresses placed side by side on the floor, a dresser, and a mirror. The other room had been the old laundry room. It was our "kitchen," with a stove and sink, table and chairs, and an old dark sideboard. We had to go downstairs for the bathroom. Each room had a gas fire in a fireplace.

I realized that I knew these streets. I knew the laundromat we had been to was five blocks away. Every two weeks or so Keith and I had carried our suitcases filled with dirty clothes down the four flights of stairs and walked to that laundromat. Once we had gone in our best clothes, I in a long black dress and Keith in a velvet suit, because everything else we owned was dirty.

I was just eighteen then. I knew exactly what I wanted to do with my life but it was scaring me: I knew I wanted to play the flute and I knew I wanted Keith. Neither of these goals received any support from my family. I don't think they knew how to support them—they made my family too uncomfortable. I come from a family of about fifty cousins all of whom went to Groton, St. Paul's, Harvard, and Yale. Like our ancestors they all became lawyers or businessmen, or married lawyers or businessmen. I wanted to play the flute. And I was in love with a man from Queens who was half Irish-Catholic, half Russian-Jewish. Who had gone to public school and the Manhattan School of Music. Who was using his classical piano training to be a rock musician and songwriter. Who had a crippled leg. Who had no money. Who I knew was a spectacular man.

We were in London because I had devised a plan: I had told my parents I wanted a year off before I started college. A six-week course at the Cordon Bleu justified my being in London. I knew all along that Keith would join me there.

We lived in a kind of stop-time then too. We knew there was a limited future in London—Keith didn't have a work permit or even a piano. But in living together we were laying a foundation for our life as a couple. We were tentatively getting to know each other away from all outside influences except those that came in the mail: worried, anxious letters from my mother and other relatives, which gave me nightmares for a few days and then were forgotten.

I was working as a maid three mornings a week, and Keith was taking tapes of his music around to record companies. In the afternoon I would play my flute in our kitchen. Sometimes I would play for Keith. We sent sightseeing. Once a week we went to the outdoor market in Soho and bought vegetables, cheese, dried beans, and bread. We drank tea and watched the sun go down. At night we lit the gas fire in the bedroom and stuffed clothes in the spaces around the door frame to keep the drafts out and the heat in. The housekeeper downstairs thought we were crazy for using the gas fires so much. But we couldn't imagine going to bed and not being able to comfortably lie naked on top of the sheets in the middle of the night, making love and talking.

We walked all over London that fall. Our steps fit. Keith's crippled leg was the permanent result of his polio, but it didn't seem to hold him back. When I had first gone out with him I had been insecure about my pace with him. By the time we were in London I knew how to match my stride to his. I knew when he needed to lean on me, when to offer him my arm going down stairs. And I could lean on him too. He had seemed endlessly strong to me then.

That November we cooked a Thanksgiving turkey for Keith's sister-in-law's cousin and her boyfriend. I remember putting the food outside on the windowsill because we didn't have a refrigerator. We bought some candles. Keith put candles everywhere: in dishes on the floor, on the mantel, on the windowsills. The candles and the gas fires were the only light. In candlelight the two rooms were transformed, in the same way a stage is transformed when the house lights go down and the stage lights go up. Our two rooms were no longer someone else's storage rooms—

they were the stage for our life, and they were beautiful. The flickering shadows and warm firelight created a physical representation of what our living together meant to us—a magical space that was both a sanctuary from our doubts and a starting point for our dreams.

We were thrilled to be together in a home that was ours, having escaped (so we thought) our pasts. We were excited that we finally had a chance to do things our own way. That Thanksgiving Keith had said to our guests, "Betsy and I get along so well because we're both the misfits in our families." We all laughed then, but I see the implications now.

Now, fourteen years later, I can see what Keith meant to me at that stage of my life. He was an escape from the world of Ivy League colleges, stories of my ancestors' accomplishments, and remarks tinged with suspicion about anything that had to do with self-expression or, God forbid, vanity. An escape from a world where the emphasis was on external achievement void of any hint of introspection. I felt Keith had saved me from the world of unspoken emotions, a world where you could cry and tear your hair out all afternoon alone in your room and no one would take notice as long as you showed up on time for dinner.

I remember when I was fifteen years old lying on my bed picturing how my life would be if it "worked out." I saw four years at college, then a respectably handsome husband, then a house in the country with, perhaps, an apartment in the city. Then the husband faded out and children appeared—not a group of individuals but a noisy herd. I saw myself making an endless stream of peanut-butter-and-jelly sandwiches, wrapping them in waxed paper to be put in picnic baskets and taken on sailing picnics, to swimming pools, or on hikes up mountains. Not a bad life, I told myself, but horrifying in its predictability. I felt it was a life that had been created by someone other than me— my only role was to assume my place in it. At fifteen I thought a life was something you were born into. I didn't know it was something you could create. I didn't know there were alternatives.

Until the next year when I met Keith. Keith was obsessed with creating his life. Perhaps it was because he had almost lost his life to polio. Perhaps it was because of a need to express his musical talents. Now I see that perhaps it was also because of his need to get away from the emotional and physical pain of his childhood. Whatever the reasons, he was hell-bent on creating a life built on self-expression and artistic excellence. A life in which fear was to be overcome and pride was to be nurtured, introspection indulged and performance respected. I looked at Keith and saw a man who never shied away from the flamboyant, was not afraid of extremes. Confused and floundering in my own life at sixteen, I was drawn to him like iron to a magnet.

We had met at our friends Virginia and Eric Hailey's Manhattan apartment. Keith, just out of music school, was temporarily living in their maid's room while he tried to get his career off the ground. One night I came to babysit for their children. We sat in the kitchen and talked and talked—physically drawn to each other but shyly keeping our distance. ("He's so sophisticated," I thought. "What could he see in me?")

Our relationship solidified the next year when Keith had his own tiny studio apartment on Fiftieth Street and Tenth Avenue. Two songwriters lived in a carriage house across the courtyard from his apartment. Sometimes we went to visit them and listen to their work. Sometimes we'd go to visit the Haitian superintendent in his ground-floor shop where he sold voodoo objects. He'd show us necklaces and wooden statues—tell us what they symbolized, what powers they had. Keith's world seemed endlessly exotic to me. By January of that year, my senior year in high school, I was regularly cutting school and spending days

with him in his apartment—writing term papers in my underwear on a typewriter at the foot of his bed.

The winter we were in England I did my Christmas shopping
on Oxford Street. It was my first Christmas away from home
and I was feeling fragile and a little homesick. And the weather
was perpetually damp and misty and gray. I walked back to
Seymour Street, up the stairs to our two rooms, and there was
Keith with a small Christmas tree. He put it on the sideboard.
I sat down and took out the stiff, wired wrapping ribbon I had
bought and bent it into ornaments—circles and stars.

That Christmas I bought Keith a butterfly made of sequins
from a woman in Soho. I sewed it onto the jacket of his velvet
suit. Keith's best man wore that jacket with the butterfly at our
wedding two years later. I had sewed it on very carefully.
Everything I did that fall and winter was careful. Attentive,
careful, devoted. I have always thought of that time as magical.
Tentative and provisional as it was, it was specially blessed. For
we were secure in our love even while being unsure of the world,
unsure of our future. We were purposeful, and we ached for
each other.

I had been frightened to leave that time too.

But I didn't think of those things that afternoon fourteen
years later on Oxford Street. I couldn't think. All I felt was my
insides being sucked out of me.

Here I was packing to go back to our home, to our baby,
but this time my homesickness couldn't be appeased. I was going
through the motions of getting ready to go home yet getting
more desperately homesick by the minute. The home I longed
for, the life I had lived, no longer existed—and never would
again. Although I wasn't consciously aware of it then, somewhere inside I knew it.

*   *   *

The morning of our flight home I packed our bags. Tipped the help at the hotel. Arrived at the hospital right on schedule. It was all going fine. Robert was with us, making sure that we had everything we needed.

But watching Keith get dressed sickened me with fear—he was so weak. I had to put Keith's shoes on for him, buckle his belt. Pushing him in his wheelchair to say good-bye to the nurses was haunting. The nurses were warm and sweet but their eyes looked upset, as if they knew they were saying good-bye to a doomed and dying man.

The car service had sent a beautiful Bentley to take us to the airport, but Keith, who would have enjoyed it before, hardly noticed. We drove along streets that I had walked in various states of shock, panic, grief, love, and anger. It was peculiar to pass them, leave them, in the morning sun. I wanted to show them to Keith and say, "This is where I bought you the sandwich you wanted, that is the post office where I sent a postcard to Luke, there's the turnoff to the hotel. This is the outside of the drama." But I didn't. It would have been irrelevant to Keith. Keith was thinking his own thoughts.

We had to wait to board the plane and Keith was looking whiter by the minute. When he stood up to leave his wheelchair and walk to his seat I wished I could disappear. Anything would be better than having to see this through. Standing in the door of the plane Keith stopped. He was trying to figure out how to make his body work. He couldn't conceive of making it down the aisle to his seat. But he made it. It just took more than he thought he had. After we got Keith settled, Robert went to his seat in another section of the plane and left me and Keith alone.

The smoky air on the plane made it hard for Keith to breathe. He couldn't stop coughing. We needed to ask for oxygen.

When I got up to go to the bathroom, a stewardess took me

aside and asked what was wrong with my husband. I told her he was recovering from pneumonia, just out of the hospital. She said she had had pneumonia once. Terrible. "Here, I'll take him a bowl of hot water so he can breathe in the steam. It will help his cough." Keith spent the flight with his head under a blanket over a steaming bowl of hot water and with a tank of oxygen next to him.

Talking to that stewardess symbolized to me the real beginning of the lies—the lies we would need to get help. I had lied about Keith's condition before—to the people in the hotel who had been politely concerned, to the musicians Keith had abruptly stopped working with, to the car service and the airline. But they didn't count. They weren't an ongoing part of our lives. The flight home, however, was supposed to be a beginning: our reentry into a life where things were familiar and comfortable. Obviously the lying was coming home with us.

On the plane I started thinking about an afternoon when I had had tea alone in my hotel room. I had come back from the hospital for a nap. It was right after we had been given the O.K. for Keith to come home. He was getting stronger, and I was just beginning to realize how terrified I was of his coming home. Since I had arrived in England I had had a recurring nightmare in which I returned home and saw myself in the hall mirror of our apartment as I walked in the door with my suitcases. When I saw myself in the mirror I knew that I was alone, that Keith wasn't ever going to walk in the door with me again. I always woke up crying.

That afternoon at the hotel I finally knew that wasn't going to happen and I was glad. But the relief was much less complete than I had expected. Who was this man I was going to go home with? He didn't look like himself. He could hardly speak. (His vocal chords had been damaged by all the tubes.) And all the doctors said that things were only going to get worse. Even as

I was having these awful thoughts, thoughts that to me seemed disloyal to Keith, I was enjoying being alone. I was thinking: This is the last time that I will be alone for a long time. I was enjoying being alone so much—too much, I feared.

But I had forgotten how many ways there are of being alone. I felt terribly alone on that plane with Keith sitting next to me. Though I held his hand under his lap blanket, we didn't talk. It wasn't because talking made him cough; it was because we didn't know what to say. No words seemed appropriate. I was afraid of what was waiting in New York but I couldn't articulate my fears. I was desperately anxious to see Luke again, but if I acknowledged how much I had missed him I'd have to acknowledge the magnitude of what had happened. My feelings all seemed contradictory, I couldn't make any sense of them—and I knew enough not to want to try.

We arrived home the Tuesday night before Thanksgiving. Coming home, walking in our front door, we unsuspectingly entered a vacuum of despair and hopelessness. Pat had met us at the airport. She and Keith embraced each other. They cried. When we finished with customs we got into the limo Pat had waiting—and proceeded to get stuck in traffic. Everything stopped, the traffic and our conversation. For hours we sat in silence. When we finally arrived at our apartment building Keith put one arm around his sister's shoulders and his other arm around mine. We shuffled to the elevator. Robert followed with our bags. Silence. The elevator door opened and there was Luke in his grandmother's arms. Luke looked at Keith and me and turned away. He cried when my mother tried to hand him to me. At that moment it seemed as though the bottom fell out of the whole situation. I felt there was no foundation to build on, no reason to make an effort—hopeless.

Robert put down our bags and left. Pat said good-bye and left. My mother took her bags and left. We were left alone. Keith lay on our bed too exhausted to get undressed. I busied myself with putting Luke to bed. And while I was doing so I realized there was a reason to keep trying to go on. Even though he looked at me with confusion in his eyes, he felt blissfully familiar in my arms.

But our apartment didn't feel familiar. Our home didn't feel as though it was mine anymore: it was filled with signs of someone else running the house—different food in the refrigerator, the furniture slightly rearranged. Now that I was home I couldn't relax. It was as if I had been trapped in a nightmare that I had thought I would wake up from when I got home, only to find that I had waked up to a worse nightmare. Now I knew there was no way out.

That first night home I think I went crazy. Just when Keith was at his lowest, so tired he couldn't move, I fell apart, sobbing. Looking at Keith lying in bed staring at the ceiling with a face of stone, his crutches leaning against the wall, I sobbed myself to sleep. And then I got up at 5 A.M. to clean the apartment, put my mark on it, obliterate the past month. I found a folder my mother had put by our bed filled with information about AIDS. Pamphlets hidden out of sight in a large envelope. Discussions of "safe sex," how the virus is transmitted, how to offer support to a "friend with AIDS." What was this doing in my home? My husband needed oxygen on the plane and I came home to pamphlets next to our bed about the safety of golden showers. Courtesy of my mother! I threw that into the trash can along with all the other signs of someone else's having been in our home.

I was possessed. I went shopping for Thanksgiving dinner. My mother came to help. Luke shrieked when he saw her. I guess he thought that her presence meant I was going to go away again. I hardly remember Keith that day. He stayed in bed—in our bed, which was in the middle of the living room, between the piano and the kitchen door. All this bustle and my craziness going on around him. I think I pretended he wasn't there. Bustling around as if to spite him.

I felt that there had to be the smell of turkey in our home on Thanksgiving. There always had been. Or had been since six years before, a year when we had had family commitments Thanksgiving Day, and had decided to have our own Thanksgiving dinner with friends the preceding night. We called it our Lost Souls' or Wayward Thanksgiving, because we invited anyone we knew who didn't have a place to go or who was feeling ambivalent about where he or she was going. It became a tradition. An orgy of martinis and wine and food. Cooking in our little galley kitchen. Everyone appreciative and festive. At one in the morning when our friends had left, the dirty dishes would be practically trailing out the kitchen door. Keith and I would organize them before we went to bed. Thanksgiving morning we would drink lots of espresso, get in a cab, and go uptown to watch the parade. Then we would go home and drink Bloody Marys, maybe do some dishes, and fix ourselves turkey sandwiches before proceeding on to whatever family events we'd promised to attend. My favorite Thanksgivings were those when we didn't have any commitments at all Thanksgiving Day. Then we'd fill our plates with sandwiches and leftover pie and get in bed for the rest of the day with some champagne.

I just couldn't see all that stopping so suddenly, so completely. So I cooked a turkey and Keith ate on a tray in bed, Luke in his high chair, I at the table. Going through the motions. Keith couldn't eat. I didn't want to eat. Luke was trying to figure out what was going on.

Pathetic, I guess. I so desperately wanted to make our home cozy and secure. It just couldn't happen then. So I did the dishes. And when Luke had gone to bed I scrubbed the kitchen floor with Clorox. Our kitchen was about three feet away from Keith in bed. The smell of Clorox probably overshadowed that of the turkey. The same way my anger was overshadowing any loving emotions I might have had. As if I wasn't going to nurture Keith, I was going to scrub him away. Attack with sterility if we couldn't be fertile.

It was insanity.

Keith's temperature stayed below 100 the first forty-eight hours we were home, but then it started to hover between 101 and 102. We knew we needed a doctor. We never wanted to see Dr. Cohen again, but now that we'd given up on Keith's regular doctor because of the penicillin mistake, she was the only doctor we knew. In England they had said that the best thing we could do was to get in touch with the gay community, that they were the only ones who were on top of things. I called the Gay Men's Health Crisis and they recommended Dr. Davis. I called his office but his line was out of order. Didn't inspire much confidence.

The Friday after Thanksgiving we knew that Keith needed a doctor immediately. His fever was up and he was having trouble breathing. Dr. Davis's phone was still out of order. We were left with Dr. Cohen. She was out of town so I had to speak to the doctor covering for her. He said that Keith should go to the emergency room at NYU Medical Center. Smelly, crowded, rude, noisy. They tested Keith's blood gases and x-rayed his lungs. Said his lungs were all right but he should be admitted to the hospital so they could do tests to determine what was causing the fevers. We couldn't do it—not that hospital, not with those doctors. I hated Dr. Cohen. She had misdiagnosed Keith, not to mention how callously cheerful she had sounded when I called her after hearing that Keith had been admitted to the hospital in London. How could I allow her to take care of Keith, in that hospital? I hated it there. I hated the way the interviewing nurse in the emergency room drew the curtains on our cubicle as soon as I said that Keith had AIDS. Both exhausted, Keith sick, we went home.

The next morning, Saturday, Keith woke up feeling better, his temperature normal. Perhaps he would be all right. As I was giving him his breakfast tray Luke came and stood next to the bed. He had refused to get close to Keith since we had come home. I think he was frightened by Keith—confused and frightened by the change in his father. But that morning, with a very serious face for a one-and-a-half-year-old, he stood near Keith and stared at him. Then he went back to his room and returned with a book. He climbed into bed next to Keith and started showing *Goodnight Moon* to him. He was saying hello to Keith, and with his doing so some of the tension in the household was relieved.

At around noon Keith's fever started to climb and the tension returned. We knew we had to go to the hospital. We decided to try Dr. Davis's number once more. Someone picked up. I explained that my husband was back from England, that he had just gotten over PCP, that he was having fevers, that we didn't have a doctor. Dr. Davis said that he'd take on a new patient. He said Keith needed a workup to find out what was causing the fevers. He told us to meet him at St. Margaret's Medical Center's emergency room at two.

I remember how relieved I was that someone was telling us what to do. We needed to be somewhere at a specific time.

Pat and her husband, Larry, drove us. St. Margaret's emergency room was brisk and cold, but seemed more efficient than NYU's. They put Keith in a cubicle to wait until Dr. Davis arrived to see him. I was filling out forms when he came. When

I had finished I went into the cubicle and shook his hand. He was telling Keith why he had to be in the hospital, what tests they needed to do. He wasn't exactly Marcus Welby—he looked so young and pixyish and gay, and his bleached hair was more orange than blond. But he gave the impression of being very smart and quick. On top of things. And I was very, very impressed that while he talked he held Keith's hand and occasionally stroked his forehead.

It was late evening when Keith finally got a room. By then he was delirious with fever. A maintenance man walked into the room to check the heat and Keith thought he was a nurse. "Nurse, nurse, help me. My fever is very high." Waiting for a nurse, waiting for some Tylenol, waiting for the thermal blanket machine. In England everyone had been attentive; here they didn't seem to care. I left as soon as Keith was relatively comfortable. Not thinking. As usual, trying desperately hard not to think.

I remember talking to Keith on the phone every night during that period, usually after having spent the evening at the hospital. And then I'd have to talk to relatives too. Suddenly there were so many calls to make every night. At least the numbers were handy: while we were in London my mother had made a list of friends and relatives and had taped it by the phone. When Keith came home and noticed it, he called it "the funeral list."

If felt much harder having Keith in the hospital in New York than in England. I had come home, but it was a different home than the one I'd consoled myself with in my mind. The set was the same, but the action wasn't. In London I could always think that when we got home everything would be all right. That we'd go back to how we were before. Now that we were home I knew that was impossible. I had no illusions to comfort me.

Keith was still fighting for his life. Coming home hadn't solved anything.

And there were all the explanations that had to be made. In London nobody knew us. But now I had to try to account for the present situation to people who were part of the scenario we had left a month ago—and try to explain it to myself. I alternated between the shock and grief of those who knew (family) and the confusion and uncertainty of those to whom I lied (almost everyone else).

Every night when I came home from the hospital the doorman would ask how Keith was, when he was coming home. I had told him that Keith had had a relapse caused by the strain of traveling. Then I would get upstairs and my grandmother would call. Her voice was always filled with love and concern: "We all love Keith. He is a very important part of the family; it would be terrible if anything happened to him." I was touched. I appreciated her saying that.

Keith's paternal great-grandfather had immigrated from Russia in the 1890s. A few years after his immigration he had gone back to Russia to get his wife and children, only to abandon them when they arrived in New York. Keith's grandfather and great aunts and uncles grew up in an orphanage. Each child had to make his or her own way. Keith's maternal grandmother had come from Ireland to work as a servant to an American family. Later, she worked as a maid to support her four children, after her husband left her (left her or was killed by the Ku Klux Klan on a trip to Texas; the story was always vague and uncertain). Keith's mother was working as a receptionist at Arthur Murray's Dance Studio when she met Keith's father—then a dance instructor, later a photographer.

Although his family often put Keith in a rage, and did some things that I thought were strange (such as not getting together on holidays or acknowledging the children's birthdays), I was intrigued by them. At seventeen I had thought: My family is a stiff fossil of the American dream, Keith's family is the real thing.

We used to joke about our families together (Keith did great imitations of my relatives), but for each of us the other's family held considerable attraction. Keith was drawn to the rituals of my family and the security they represented: toasts before Christmas dinner, long summer vacations in a family compound. He was impressed with my family's accomplishments. Keith saved the newspaper clippings when my uncle was chosen as special prosecutor in the Watergate affair; he memorized my family tree. While I had a tendency to let the family silver tarnish, Keith kept it polished.

Looking back I see that it is no small accomplishment that each of us became accepted into the other's family, as individuals and as a couple, and later, with the birth of Luke, as a family ourselves.

My immediate family was concerned and supportive. I appreciated their concern but it hurt me to see it. Their sympathy was a constant reminder to me that this was a terrible crisis, a tragedy that required their involvement. My sister Ann, who had come to town for the holidays, was spending her evenings babysitting for Luke while I was at the hospital.

When I came home Luke would be in the bath with her two-year-old son, Jesse, Keith's and my godchild, and her newborn would be curled up asleep on a blanket on the bed in the living room. There was often dinner on the stove. Our apartment was so warm after the hospital I couldn't fit the two things together: our home and the hospital. Then Ann would leave with her babies and Luke would go to sleep and I would get into bed alone. Suddenly I would realize how desperately I missed Keith.

But I couldn't cry. I would lie there staring at the ceiling and try to hear Luke breathing in his crib.

In the mornings I took Luke to his play group at Theresa's. I'd meet the other mothers on the stairs. Listen to them saying how wonderful it was that Keith was home, that he was all right. Make up lies. Try to look as if I too thought everything was great. Try to smile while I knew that Keith was getting ready for a CAT scan, a spinal tap, a bone-marrow tap—horrible hospital technology looking for horrible things.

Although to me it felt harder to have Keith in the hospital in New York than in London, I knew it was better for Keith. He felt safer on his own turf, so to speak. He had visitors. Virginia and Eric (the couple that had introduced us to each other) came to see him one afternoon.

Keith was so pleased to see them. To both Keith and me they had often been like surrogate parents. Virginia walked into his hospital room and gave Keith a huge hug and said, "I am not going to let you go. I am not going to let you leave this earth." I stiffened, felt myself withdraw from the scene. I was confused by my reaction—and slightly ashamed of it. I was jealous. Virginia had acknowledged that Keith was in danger of dying while being warm and affectionate. How was she able to do that? I wondered.

Keith's parents came into town from Long Island. They had lunch with Luke and me before they went to the hospital. Strange to have my in-laws in our apartment without Keith. I felt awkward around them. We had never talked about important things together and it was obvious that none of us knew how to start now. Since Keith's illness Pat had done most of the communicating with them.

I couldn't tell what they were thinking, but it seemed to me they acted as if they didn't realize how serious this was, or perhaps they did and they didn't know how to deal with it, what to do.

Keith's father gave me a check for $1,000. At least that was some acknowledgment of the seriousness of the situation. Keith's older brother, Michael, arrived. I left the room to put Luke down for his nap, and when I came back Michael was in tears and nobody was talking.

Pat invited Luke and me to have dinner and light the candles on the first night of Hanukkah with her, Larry, and their son, Brandon. Luke was happy playing with Brandon. I remember looking around and thinking how cozy and complete it was in their home. I felt so lacking, so needy. Lacking Keith. This was a family celebration, and I didn't know what had happened to mine.

Keith was treated with Septra. The fevers went away. The tests didn't turn up anything. After two and a half weeks, Dr. Davis told him he could go home.

Before Keith left St. Margaret's, the hospital gave him some written material on living with AIDS. Disinfect any spills of body fluids with bleach and water. Never share a razor or toothbrush. Wash dishes in the hottest water possible. Let them air-dry because dish towels and hand towels harbor bacteria. (Rolls of paper towels are all over the apartment now. When Keith washes his hands he dries them with a paper towel, then he turns off the faucet with it so he won't pick up any of our germs.)

Dr. Davis also talked with Keith about taking care of himself. No raw vegetables or unpeeled fruits—microorganisms on the peels could be dangerous to him. Stay away from animals. Avoid public transportation; never take the subway. Never have sex when I am menstruating. Always use condoms, and withdraw before ejaculating.

I was with Keith when Dr. Davis stood at the foot of his bed and rattled off these guidelines. It was oddly exhilarating being given this information. Keith was being told how to live, not how to die; being told that he might, with some modifications, have a fairly normal life. No one had even implied such a thing to us before.

After Dr. Davis left the room, however, I found the memory of his cheery voice a little bizarre. He had been talking about taking subways and having sex to a man who could hardly walk to the bathroom. Keith and I were both silent. I suppose we were thinking about the reality of the present, compared to which normal life seemed a distant abstraction.

Dr. Davis said he wanted to see Keith every two weeks. He put Keith on naltrexone to boost his immune system. And on Fansidar to keep PCP from returning.

Naltrexone is a new drug (or new to treating AIDS). There are only two drugstores in all New York that prepare it. One is in Brooklyn. The one we go to is in the East Village.

While Keith was in the hospital I had prayed for him to come home. But when he came home all the anger came back. I wanted Keith home, not this sickly, silent man. I felt I was suddenly living with a very old, old man, a different man from the one in my thoughts.

I remember John Lande telling me to let my anger out. I remember screaming and hitting that orange-vinyl-covered chair with my fists when I had that first session with him. "Hit something. Beat the pillows at night. Let your anger out every night," he had told me. But now I don't want to let my anger out. I need to keep it. It's my strength. I want to use it. I want to use it to get through each day until we've gotten through enough days to put England behind us and all the things the doctors said are proven wrong.

This anger gets me up each morning. If it went away I don't know how I'd find the energy to change Luke's diapers, take him out to play, buy the groceries. And I'm scared of the feelings I would have if I let go of my anger.

In the mornings I wake up disoriented. It isn't until the day has progressed, gathered its own momentum, that I feel present. Because by then some little memories have been stored up: the memory of Luke getting into bed with Keith in the morning, the memory of Keith smiling when I bring Luke home from play group, flushed and happy in his snowsuit. But where am I in these mental snapshots? In the kitchen making breakfast. Struggling to get Luke out of his snowsuit while he protests and wiggles.

What is this balancing act I have to do? I'm balancing anger and confusion against a love and appreciation more acute than I have ever felt before. There are moments when I see Keith with Luke that I feel rich and full. I should try to concentrate on them. Every night, when Luke sits on Keith's lap in the rocking chair and Keith is reading Luke his bedtime story, I feel that time has stopped. I appreciate, I am thankful. We are living as a family. For these moments life is good. We are living. We had another day. The doctors in England are crazy, they were wrong.

I hate the doctors in England for the things they said to me.

I hate them for saying that if they had known Keith had AIDS when he was admitted to the hospital they would have let him die; they wouldn't have put him on a respirator. I hate them for telling me that Keith has only six months left to live, eleven at the most.

No one is dying when he is putting his baby son to bed. Why did they say those things to me?

When the day is over I get in bed with Keith and I can't sleep.

Everyone is crazy about this disease. Each one has his or her own theories, preconceptions, opinions. I wonder what it would be like if we were told Keith had a very serious cancer and had six months to live: Would it be easier? Actually, if we could manage to stop listening to people, listening to the media, I would believe that all the unknowns about AIDS give us lots of room for hope. Because anything can happen.

But there is the stigma of AIDS to contend with as well. Only close friends and family know that Keith has AIDS. In England I made the decision not to tell anyone else because I didn't want Luke to be a victim of anyone's fears and ignorance. This catastrophic event in our lives goes unspoken so that our son won't lose a chance at getting into nursery school, so if Luke falls in the playground and is bleeding he won't be denied a hug. I have this image of Luke falling down and no one picking him up or giving him a hug because they think he's contaminated. I couldn't stand it if Luke missed a hug because of his Daddy's disease.

And, please God, if—when—Keith becomes strong enough to work again, who would hire him? Who would want to work with him?

So we're isolated and alone with our secret. And this secretiveness makes things confused, makes me feel there is something to be ashamed of. Even Dick, when he heard, said, "Luke must never know."

It seems that everyone I tell asks how Keith got AIDS. Why? What are they responding to, the disease or what it represents?

I hate being asked how Keith caught AIDS. I know part of me hates it because it is something I don't want to think about—

and if I won't ask myself how Keith got sick, how dare they ask? But it is more than that. In asking how Keith got sick I feel people are implying that there must be some way of making sense of all this. My own feeling is that nothing can explain such complete devastation of a person's life.

Sometimes I wish there was an explanation, a place to put the blame. For lack of one I find myself unable to figure out what I think. There are so many feelings, so many fears that Keith and I don't mention to each other, or to ourselves. We don't know what to say to each other, how to begin. I am angry and confused. Keith feels guilty, marked. And he is scared. We are both so scared.

We are living in a double cocoon—isolated from each other and isolated from the world. Maybe it has to be this way now. We need to find our own personal resources, our individual reserves of strength. We need to believe that Keith is going to get well. And if we are the only two people in the world who think so then we must keep our distance from everyone else.

But where are all the things that used to make us strong?

That's what I'm missing now. I'm missing feeling strong. And I'm missing feeling strong with Keith. I'm always watching now—watching Keith, watching Luke, watching Keith and Luke together, watching life, desperately trying to keep it going. I see so much now. The simplest, most mundane things break my heart. But something is gone. Something that worked between Keith and me.

I remember the summer Keith's band played at Danceteria. Keith was a success. After the performance he and I went to breakfast. We walked home with our arms around each other. The sun was just coming up. The city was quiet. Looking at each other made us smile. We were happy and proud. We felt self-contained and knowing. It was a moment when walking down the street together was more intimate than making love. Life seemed to be a condition of endless possibilities. I remember feeling blissfully content, because we had such pride, so many plans for the future, and so much happiness in the present.

I am thinking of a photograph of Keith and me taken the night of my twenty-fifth birthday. I had gone out for a drink with a friend that evening, believing that I would go home later, change out of my jeans, and go out to dinner with Keith. Instead I came home to a house full of friends. Keith had made me a surprise party. There were my classical-musician friends and my friends from the waitress job I was working a few nights a week. Keith had taken such care.

In the photograph Keith has his arm around me. We are looking at each other and smiling, beaming really. I am licking icing off my fingers. I love that picture because we are glowing. I also love that picture because it immediately followed one that someone had taken of the cake Keith had made for me and hidden on the floor of his closet: a huge, gooey cake dripping icing in the middle of his shoes. I had loved seeing that. The cake among the shoes and then Keith and me obviously enjoying each other so much. I can't think about that now. We never enjoy each other anymore.

I want Keith to put his arms around me and tell me everything will be all right, tell me to relax. But how can I expect Keith to do that for me? Keith for whom things will never be all right again?

In St. Margaret's Keith registered with the Gay Men's Health Crisis. They assigned him a buddy, Wayne. Keith had said he didn't need Wayne, he had me. (It was typical of that time that I liked hearing Keith say that. I wanted to be all he needed, even if I knew rationally that that was an impossibility.) But one day Keith called Wayne to come over and help him watch Luke so that I could go out alone and do some Christmas shopping. It made me too nervous to leave Luke and Keith alone together. I had this feeling that I had to do everything, be everything to everyone. I couldn't imagine anything working without me.

But Wayne arrived. Young, energetic, and warm. He made conversation with Keith—asked him how he was feeling, what medications he was taking. He got down on the floor to play with Luke.

I left. I can't remember where I went. I can't remember what I bought. I can't remember what presents I gave to Luke or to Keith. Maybe Keith and I didn't give each other presents. It was less than a month ago and still I can't remember. But I remember coming home later that morning.

I opened the door and saw Keith's, Luke's, and Wayne's wet boots dripping in the hall. Keith was sitting at the table. Wayne was playing with Luke on the floor. They were all flushed with fresh air. Keith said that Wayne had suggested they take a walk. It was thrilling to me that they had done that. I loved Wayne at that moment. He had scored a major victory over our defeatism. I guess I remember that scene so clearly because it fed the feeling that was growing inside me that Keith would get well. He must get well.

My memories of Christmas are scattered and vague. By then I think we had accepted things more. Or at least I acknowledged that I couldn't scrub the disease out of our house. And I saw Keith getting stronger at home and that felt good, really good. Keeping him out of the hospital, at home, became all that mattered. And seeing him with Luke.

We have some snapshots of Christmas Day: Luke opening presents, Keith and Luke playing with Luke's new toys, Keith and me in our pajamas on the floor under our Christmas tree, Christmas dinner at my parents' house. But I can't remember bringing home our Christmas tree or decorating it. I can't remember what any of it felt like.

I guess Christmas hit too many nerves. To get through it we had to pretend that everything was all right. Why can't I remember Christmas? Because half of it was a charade, and the half that wasn't was too confusing and too painful for me to take in. Right now, what little pieces I remember of Christmas I think of as being part of a dream. Like the bottle of Perrier at my parents' bar, obviously bought for Keith. When my father asked Keith what he wanted to drink, Keith asked for some scotch: "Don't worry, I'm not going to turn green."

After Christmas Keith and I started seeing a psychotherapist, Dr. Gorman, who specializes in AIDS victims. We also went to a nutritionist, and took preliminary steps toward consulting a Tibetan doctor that Keith's cousin John had told us about. I packed up a bottle of Keith's urine to be sent to India so that Tibetan doctors could analyze it and prescribe treatment.

With the possible exception of the Tibetan doctors it all seems wrong, very wrong, and even a little silly. Dr. Gorman seems fairly uninspired, although he did get Keith and me to talk to each other. The nutritionist was offensive, saying that the only AIDS patients he had who died wanted to die.

But these attempts to get help, futile or not, have helped us begin to see where we are—first steps toward acknowledging our situation. Because now we've established a routine, if you could call it a routine. More like we've settled in, tried to feel out our space, tried to get comfortable.

Without really talking about it, we've constructed a way of coping. We are coping by getting through one day at a time. It is very private. We need to isolate ourselves. That is what I am feeling now. The isolation that at other times seemed so terribly oppressive has begun, in a subtle way, to comfort us. Keith must not go into the hospital again; he must stay here, with me and Luke. When he is home we are a unit, and it is within that unit that Keith will get well.

WINTER

Yesterday my tension broke—or rather my temper broke. Everything seemed sickness, colds, and claustrophobia. Keith and I fought. Keith gets stronger and I get angrier—it's a pattern I have to figure out how to stop. Keith seems so good at being sick, quietly accepting AIDS as his fate, while I'm so bad at, so furious at, having a sick husband.

Stop. That isn't it. It's not a sick husband. That's not what I was crying about, not what I'm so angry about. It's the events in his life that led to this that make me want to scream. They seem sordid and pathetic. The age of innocence is over and the world seems crueler and sicker than I could ever have imagined. Everything seems false. And I told Keith that. Poured salt in his wounds. I said it: sordid and pathetic. I said it through my sobs.

What happened? When did Keith tell me? Did he tell me after he came home from St. Margaret's? I can't remember being close enough to him after he came home from St. Margaret's— or at any time in the period since his AIDS diagnosis—to have had this conversation. But I remember it. I just can't remember exactly when it took place.

I remember that Keith was in earnest, painfully in earnest. It was as if he were reaching for his lifeline—my acceptance. No, more than my acceptance. He was desperate for my forgiveness. And that hurt. That made me angry. Scared. No forgiveness. That's pathetic, Keith asking for forgiveness. That's Keith hating himself. I didn't want to acknowledge that there was anything to forgive.

The earnestness in Keith's voice. Heartbreaking. I remember his saying that what Pat had told me wasn't true. Yes, he had lived with a man his first year in college. He had desperately needed to move out of his parents' house and that was the only way he could figure out to do it. They didn't live together long. He hated it. He moved into a room at the Y as soon as he had the money. But when he went to Saratoga six years ago he went to see that man only to make peace with his past. He did not have sex with him.

He said that the summer he went to Saratoga he had been having anonymous sex with men. He couldn't help himself. He wanted to stop. It made him hate himself. That is why he had started therapy again. Once he had started therapy he wanted to see this man again. To put it to rest. (And he did, he said— that was the end of his sexual relations with men.)

Then I remember he started to cry. He said that he had gone to a doctor for antibiotics to take so that he wouldn't catch any disease that he could give me. He said, If only he had known. How could he have known? He didn't know. Nobody knew then.

At that moment AIDS didn't matter to me. What he had done did. How did this fit into our life? Our life as I had seen it? Why? But Keith looked so pained. Then he was sobbing. I cannot get angry at him. He is suffering. Please stop suffering, stop hating yourself, please stop hating yourself. I want you here. Stop. Just stop. It doesn't matter. Really, it doesn't matter. Please stop crying. I remember that summer. We were reckless that summer. We took each other for granted. We pushed everything to the limit. We knew we loved each other. I was staying out all night too. It was O.K. because we knew we had each other. And we always came home to each other.

As Keith told me what had happened that summer I remember having so much nostalgia for the way I had felt then. In my innocence I was sure that we had made ourselves a foundation so strong that anything could happen above the foundation and be acknowledged, laughed at, held secret or shared—it wouldn't matter. I had loved that summer while we were living it, but now it represents Keith's downfall. Now, in retrospect, I remember that he was depressed then. Looking back on it I think that maybe I stayed out all night with friends because I wanted to avoid Keith. Maybe I didn't want to see what was going on.

This is changing the way I see my past. What I thought of at the time as high-spirited recklessness I'm now being asked to see as desperation. I can't do it. It's too scary to change my memories. So I tell Keith over and over again that it doesn't matter. It's O.K. I love him.

But it doesn't feel O.K. Why did he do this? My faithful, devoted man. My proud man. My favorite. The person who inspired all the most special times in my life. My home. Why? Keith and I sat at our dining room table as he talked. I remember the sun on the wood of the table as I scratched my nails into the table's surface.

I asked Keith why. What he did didn't make sense to me. I needed to know why. I wanted to see our past and trust it. I had to be able to fit it in or I would be living with a stranger. My memories wouldn't make sense. Keith is not a gay man. If I can't trust that belief then I have to rethink, reinterpret what my memories of him and me mean. I cannot continue if I doubt them, if they are no longer valid. But I know they are valid. Otherwise I wouldn't have had the courage to ask him. Why did you do that?

And he told me. And I dug my nails into the surface of the table. He told me about the sexual abuse that had occurred when he was growing up. He was shaking. For the moment my anger dissolved. That was enough of an explanation for me.

That made sense to me. That explained why Keith was so anchored in the present—almost defiantly so—and bitter about the past.

And, most important, it made pieces of the puzzle fit into place. That summer six years ago Keith had been depressed about his career. He had been hoping to get a record contract and it had fallen through. He had tried hard and felt he had failed. I remember thinking more than once that summer that there was a streak of depression in Keith that was nothing short of desperate. He was drinking a lot, he was having nightmares, and he was losing his temper over little things.

Keith is a talented and skilled musician. He is a charismatic performer. He is, even with AIDS, an extremely handsome man. But that summer I remember it occurred to me that perhaps, in some way, Keith didn't quite believe these things about himself. I remembered he once said, "Every time I walk into a room it is a performance." Keith felt he had to create a self for the world to see. Until that summer, I had never seen the effort because the effect was so dazzling.

It was the investment of his ego in his music and performing

that made his work unique and powerful. I now see the flip side
of that—rejection was absolutely devastating to him. That summer Keith's ego was gone.

But I also remember times of incredible closeness that summer. We were separate during the days and most of the nights,
but sometimes in the early morning when the sun was coming
up we would surface from sleep and make love and hold each
other. I cannot hate Keith for what he did that summer. I loved
him and knew he loved me. I loved the way we held each other,
as if we were about to fall off a ledge. And I loved feeling that
in holding each other we would stop the fall. It is so painful
now to realize that we didn't stop it. It happened, and we didn't
even know it.

So now I understand how it is that my husband has AIDS.
Keith who I thought kept no secrets from me has finally told
me the one most devastating secret of his life.

I feel lonelier than I can ever remember feeling. Sometimes
it's as though I don't know Keith anymore. Knowing about his
past seems to have changed the present. Sometimes I still can't
help thinking about it as sordid. I don't want this as part of
my life. That's what I sometimes think: our past together is
tainted—sordid and tainted. I hate myself for thinking that.

Somewhere in me I know that knowing about the past can
make the future better. That's what sharing secrets should do.
Make us closer. Clear the slate for the future.

But we are told there isn't any future. That Keith is going
to die. Understanding the past could make Keith and me closer
and then be forgotten if it weren't for Keith's having AIDS.
AIDS is making all the wrong things larger than life. And the
good things squashed. We can't hug each other anymore.

So it ends there, in my loneliness and fury. And I start feeling that I deserve more than a husband with AIDS, money worries, and a small apartment on a noisy corner. That's what my life looks like to me now when our future is taken away.

January 24

Keith and I had a session with Dr. Gorman this morning. A relief after being up late last night, the two of us screaming at each other until the early hours of the morning. ("You don't talk to me." "How can I talk to you? You're so tense." "I'd relax if you'd talk to me." "I'm not talking when you're so angry.") Going around and around in circles.

Dr. Gorman says, "Fear and anger go hand in hand. Deal with the present. Let each other be." Easier said than done. Keith and I are both too shell-shocked by the last six months to deal with the present. Dealing with the present implies a level of acceptance Keith and I haven't reached yet.

January 28

I had been thinking that I wanted to start playing my flute again, but this morning I couldn't play, so I spent the time organizing my music. I want a clean slate, a place to go. Last night I dreamt that I took an older Luke to an orchestral concert and we sat in front of the woodwind section. I pointed out the flute player and said, "That's a flute like your Mommy used to play."

Sunday morning I took Luke up on the bus to visit Pat, Larry, and Brandon. Luke loves to ride the bus. Bloody Marys, bagels, and a short trip to the park. Visiting them reminded me of the times Luke and I visited them when Keith was in St. Margaret's and I was frightened of the future and felt like a single parent visiting a complete family. That memory was so strong that it was a surprise to have Keith walk in the door a few minutes after we got home. (He had been visiting Dick.)

An old friend of mine, David, came by and took me out for a drink. When I got home we ordered up pizza for dinner. I felt I had had a day off from the household. Sunday I slept through the night for the first time in months.

Monday Keith's brother, Michael, came to dinner. Doing the dishes I was angry and felt as if the kitchen were my secret laboratory where I turned out potions that kept everyone who entered our apartment alive and strong while I got weaker and weaker. Feeding them drains me. Lots of anger still inside. Not enough nurturing of myself. I think I still have too many fears to give up the feeling that I am the one who has to keep everything going—that if I don't keep everything going awful things will happen.

I've got to get back some feeling of my own autonomy. There are times I feel as if I'm dissolving into Keith and Luke, caring for them.

I must call Susan, the therapist I had gone to before Luke was born. I called her shortly after we got home from London, and we'd agreed to meet once I felt ready to talk. I'd put her out of my mind until now. Although most of me doesn't want to talk, I'm beginning to feel that I must, or my resentment and fear will poison me and my family.

It is bitter cold out. Keith's cold is almost gone. If it weren't for the fact that his sweat smells so funny and sweet—a smell I will never forget; it's the smell I'd first noticed in Montauk, and in London his hospital room reeked of it—he would seem perfectly well. He stopped taking the Tibetan pills that had arrived from India because he was afraid they would interfere with the Fansidar and naltrexone and says he feels stronger without them. He had taken them for a week: what the Tibetans call a precious pill last Saturday and Wednesday, and little brown pills on the days in between. John is calling India to see what they say about mixing them with Western drugs.

February 8

Keith went to Dr. Davis and got a good report. His white blood count is at 3,300—up from 1,000 when he entered St. Margaret's. That afternoon Keith went to see our new accountant. Depressing news: estimated we owe $13,000 this year, which is at the moment everything we have in the bank.

So trapped by circumstances: Keith's illness and our finances and the unknown future. Not knowing if and how Keith will work is a heavy worry. Dr. Gorman keeps feeding us the perspective of infinite possibilities for improvement. He talks about changing our priorities, reworking our communication with outsiders, discovering our needs and meeting them—as if all these things will lead to some sort of answer. So far it only sounds good. It doesn't get rid of the panic I feel when I think of the future.

I needed to get out of the house. I took Luke on a bus ride across town: Luke's latest passion is buses.

I like Dr. Gorman's emphasis on learning how to relate to the outside world, and beginning to express our feelings, because I feel I am struggling with so many feelings of isolation—and a lot of uncertainty—when it comes to how Keith and I can fit into the workings of the everyday world. I hear the words "My husband has an incurable illness" in my mind as if I am trying to get used to them, practicing so that one day I may be able to say them out loud. I always seem to hear them at the strangest times, as when I'm walking Luke to Theresa's or shopping at the grocery store. They make me feel powerless and frustrated and scared. It is going to be a long time before I can say them to anyone but myself.

At our last session Keith told Dr. Gorman about trying to get home from doing an errand uptown in rush hour the other day. He said the streets were crowded, everyone was rushing, the bus didn't come and he couldn't get a taxi. He said he felt so sick and dizzy that he wanted to just sit down on the curb and cry because he couldn't manage anymore. For Keith, watching the world of the healthy passing him by, the feeling of isolation must be even stronger than it is for me.

But, while I am beginning to have moments of feeling frustrated by our isolation, Keith wants it. He finds security in it. He told Dr. Gorman that during the holidays we gave ourselves permission to let our family life and health be the foremost priority in our lives and it felt pretty good. It felt as though life had purpose and importance. He doesn't feel the underside of the isolation—the stifling—which I am beginning to feel.

This feeling of isolation is so strong. Not only do I feel isolated from the outside world, but I also feel isolated from Luke and Keith by the enormity of the emotions I cannot express. When we are comfortable, when the day is over, if Keith is feeling all right, I lie in bed and feel as if I am floating above the events in my life. Floating, never connecting. My feelings have no place to settle, no expression that has any consequence.

I am furious at life so I lose my temper and shout and scream and then collect myself. I turn to Luke and say, "Anger all gone" and give him a hug. (But it isn't gone, I've just got it under control.) If I feel panicky about Keith's health I pour more wheat germ into his pancakes. If I look at Keith bathing Luke and pray for our future I keep it to myself. If I wake at night and see Keith sitting up in bed, staring into the darkness, see his fear and begin to feel my own, I reach out and tentatively touch his shoulder. He doesn't respond. Nothing comes to a conclusion, a resolution.

February 11

Had my first session with Susan this morning. First session since Keith got sick, I mean. I told her the uncertainty of the situation was hard for me. How much time does Keith have? What's going to happen to him? It's not like cancer, a disease whose progress doctors know a lot about. Her response was sympathetic, but I cried tears of panic and guilt when she said, "You must wish that if Keith is going to die he would get it over with." I felt so guilty for ever having thought that. It wasn't the first time I had thought it: I had thought it when the English doctors were telling me that Keith had six months left to live. It really didn't seem to help when I put my feelings into words because I felt so guilty about them.

Last night as we were getting into bed Keith said he was upset and needed to talk. And we did talk. For the first time Keith opened up to me about being sick. Not about how he got AIDS, or the circumstances leading up to those events, but how he feels now, how he feels about the present. Keith is very frightened of ever having to go back in the hospital. He is also uncertain and apprehensive about what it will be like to work again. Will he be able to? He desperately wants to be able to be creative and productive. He said that he feels like dressing in robes—a symbol to tell everyone that his life has changed, forcing them to see that, without telling them he has AIDS.

After we talked I felt closer to Keith than I had at any time since I sat beside his hospital bed in London. For the first time in months I remembered again how at our best we've always felt that we didn't need anything more than each other.

I remember Keith saying to me when I was about eighteen

that he and I could move mountains together. I want to never stop believing that.

I went to sleep thinking the words "Betsy and Keith, Betsy and Keith." I felt as though I had all at once remembered all the eras in our life together and I was holding them as I was holding Keith. With such a past there has to be a future: For the first time in many months our past seems like a foundation.

February 13

Keith felt dizzy and weak this afternoon. He had gone to buy an answering machine. He got so dizzy on the street that he stopped making sense . . . and then he wondered how he would ever be able to function in the professional world. He was very dizzy and nauseated this evening and we both got scared. But he is sleeping peacefully now.

February 15

Friday was the first day I've been out with Keith that I forgot he was sick. It was the first really big snowstorm of the winter. Rachel came to visit. It was the first time I'd seen her since London and I was afraid of her treating me like a victim, a source of worry and reason for concern. But she didn't. Keith, Luke, Rachel, and I went to buy Luke boots and then we walked in the snow to the Empire Diner. Had hot rum and cider and then walked home. Luke was thrilled with the snow. We arrived back home flushed with the cold, feeling relaxed and sleepy.

Keith woke up the next morning feeling awful: fever of 102. I had been vaguely aware of his restlessness and the heat of his fever in my sleep. Dr. Davis thinks it is the flu because it came on so suddenly. I'm refusing to worry, probably being almost overly blasé.

* * *

In a bad mood all evening because I met our neighbor Christian in the hall. We were gossiping about the building and he said that Jack, another neighbor of ours, died this weekend of AIDS. I pretended that my knowledge of and concern about AIDS was the same as his, straight out of the *New York Times*. It upset me and I didn't tell Keith because he had a fever and felt achy and dizzy.

Sometimes I wish people would just leave us alone. I want to remember what I felt in England when I was praying that Keith would be able to go home: that once we got there we would have the whole universe behind our front door.

February 17

Went out to dinner with my friend Mary last night. A tequilaed Mexican dinner. I told her how Keith caught AIDS. Mary's my oldest friend and one of the very few people I've told. It was nice, confiding in a woman friend, but I came home vaguely disappointed. Disappointed because telling her the story did not take the pain away. I want someone to tell me that it is all going to be all right. That it will go away.

I know that isn't going to happen.

February 19

Keith and I made the mistake of watching two AIDS specials on TV the last two nights. Monday night the show was laughable and stupid. Last night's show on Channel Thirteen was scary. Horrifying to see healthy-looking men speak to the camera and then learn that they have since died. Keith broke down and sobbed about his fear of dying. It was heartbreaking. I comforted him as best I could, then I couldn't sleep.

We've been talking about who we should appoint as Luke's guardians when Keith has his will drawn up at the GMHC next week. They are abbreviated conversations. I think my brain shuts down on the subject. I tell myself it is a ritual that we have to go through, a ritual that will never have practical implications. I leave the decision making up to Keith. I cannot acknowledge the fact that Keith may die, much less the possibility that I could too.

I can't sleep at night. I walk from room to room, or I lie on the couch in the bedroom sipping vodka.

Eight years ago there was a second-hand mattress on this bedroom floor. A wooden milk crate was our bedside table, with a $5 lamp from Lamston's on it. We didn't even have curtains on the windows. Six years ago we bought a queen-size mattress and frame on sale at Macy's and our bedside tables were cartons of Keith's unsold records covered with blue fabric, but we still had no curtains. The sounds of traffic on Eighth Avenue and the subway vibrations through the floor, not to mention the sirens and street fights, often made it difficult to sleep.

But back then we usually went to sleep when the city did, about 3 or 4 A.M., after the night traffic had quieted and before the garbage trucks began their rounds. We talked into the night. We listened to tapes—Keith's music, a performance of mine, a performance of his. We discussed them. We went out and explored the city. Came home with friends and drank and talked. Sleep was irrelevant.

Then I got pregnant. Keith was making money. I had a steady word-processing job to supplement Keith's income and what I made from teaching and performing. The records were thrown out, although we kept a few for posterity. There was a white changing table against one wall and a child's wardrobe Keith had designed against another. And a cradle next to our bed.

Now our bed is in the living room, between the piano and the kitchen door. Luke's crib is in the bedroom, with his changing table and the wardrobe and the old living-room couch. There are blue flowered curtains on the windows lined with sound-proof padding.

At three in the afternoon when I stand in the bedroom door-way it is so quiet I can hear two people breathing. This is what I want to remember—the sound of my baby and his father breathing: Luke napping in his crib and Keith napping on the couch. Keith is wearing a headset connected to his Walkman. He fell asleep listening to a Louise Hay tape, trying to meditate away his illness, picturing his white blood cells multiplying and the AIDS virus dying.

Now it is three in the morning. I'm still listening to my baby and his father breathing, but now I'm thinking about Luke calling out for his Daddy when Keith was in the hospital and Keith looking so determined while trying to meditate away his illness. I must lie down and try to sleep. It is too quiet in here. Keith and I could always sleep if we were drunk or exhausted. Now I am both. But I feel like I will never sleep again.

February 22

Thursday evening Keith and I went to the movies. It felt great, going out on a date together.

Friday evening Michael Callen came over. Several years ago Keith had been the musical director for Michael's cabaret act. We hadn't seen him for a couple of years, although we had heard through mutual acquaintances that he had AIDS. I thought it would help Keith if he got in touch with a person with AIDS—especially someone he knows. Keith finally called Michael and the two of them went out for a drink.

I was so glad to see Keith with someone he might be able to talk to. And it was good for me to see Michael, too—he was reassuring and supportive. He confirmed my hunch that each case of AIDS is different: Michael's most serious hospitalization was for shingles (apparently they can be very serious when they appear above the waist). He has stopped taking naltrexone because it upset his stomach. Now he doesn't take any medications except antibiotics when he feels an infection coming on.

He said that when he was first diagnosed he went to a support group. The focus of the group was on preparing to die— he was the only member of the group who focused on survival. He said that is now changing, that he has seen people cope in both extremes: extreme denial and extreme despair, with neither extreme working.

Michael told Keith that if he survives AIDS he will feel that it was the best thing that could have happened to him in terms of making him appreciate every moment of his life. I can sort of understand that feeling. I know that those occasional moments of happiness with Keith and Luke which now seem so poignant would once have been taken for granted. Yes, I do appreciate more. But I'm a long way from thinking AIDS is the best thing that could have happened to us. And Keith is even further away than I am from feeling that. Still, it was good to hear someone talk about AIDS without the usual gloom and doom. Michael's optimism was especially helpful to Keith. Keith has been making phone calls to reestablish professional contacts, getting ready to work again. Michael helped him feel that yes, of course he will be able to work again.

February 23

I have a really bad cold. I'm wondering where my desire to care for myself is, where my pride is hiding.

I am thinking of Susan's suggestion of "neutralizing" myself from Keith: if he is in pain it doesn't mean that I have to be, if he is happy it doesn't mean that I can't be upset. Keith and I were so intertwined in the past: if he was troubled I should be troubled, if he was sick, I must be sick. Now he is sick and I am well; so many patterns of relating and ways of envisioning our marriage have changed—have to change. I think I have a deep-seated fear that if I am strong and independent while Keith is ill everything will fall apart. And yet I know I have to be strong or things really will fall apart.

Keith is living in fear of the next major illness, the next bout of PCP. In the meantime it's impossible for him to enjoy this respite because he's so busy taking care of the little inconveniences, discomforts, irritants that are constantly reminding him that he is sick—the muluscomes on his penis, the thrush in his mouth, the seborrhea on his scalp and eyebrows, the athlete's foot that he says itches so badly it hurts.

He has medications for all these things, and they help, but to get himself ready to meet the world, to get so he feels he has some control over his body, takes so long. It isn't just a morning shower and deodorant—he has creams and jellies and pills. It takes a lot to feel he can go out and be on equal terms with healthy people. It wears him down. I wonder if he ever really feels that he's the equal of a healthy person. No wonder he is so nervous about starting work next week, no wonder a part of him wants to retreat and live his life in our own private world.

It's cozy and secure in our home. Luke helps make it that way for us. His latest passion is popcorn. He and Keith went to buy a popcorn maker on Saturday. Luke loves watching it pop. I love watching Keith make it with him, and Luke's excitement. Luke and Keith are like two peas in a pod when it comes to enjoying life.

F e b r u a r y   2 6

Keith had his first business meeting today about a spec for L'Oreal. He has to write something to be recorded on Friday in an all-day session. Two weeks ago I would have been scared; now I'm anxiously curious to see how he deals with the pressure, phone calls, and long hours, not to mention bullshit.

I am thinking/hoping Keith's working will take some of the pressure off me in terms of his needing my support, or lessen the feeling he has that I don't give him enough because nothing I do takes away the pain of our situation. I suspect that a lot of his pain comes from his hurt pride. I'm hoping that going back to work will restore his self-esteem.

F e b r u a r y   2 7

Today we had a wonderfully cozy, snowy morning. Theresa canceled because of the snow, so I took Luke out for a walk. I loved seeing him all bundled up with snowflakes on his cheeks. When we got home he and Keith played with the set of child-size musical instruments Keith had bought him a few days ago. Keith played the piano, Luke banged on his tambourine.

F e b r u a r y   2 8

Keith is at his first all-day recording session. I came home from taking Luke to Theresa's to a sunny, clean, *empty* apartment and refused to worry. The quiet and aloneness were like magic. There is so much banging away in my brain that needs to spill out onto a clean, blank surface. Took a shower, wandered around, and felt like hugging myself.

I took out my flute to practice. Wondered why I did, since

there isn't anything to prepare for. I used to feel so driven to practice in the past, needed to feel on top of my technique. I'm certainly not on top of it now. There are no melodies in my head, no interpretations. I am just playing the notes. But I don't care. I need to do this. Because while I am playing all I am thinking about is the notes. And while I am playing I feel comfortable and at home.

When Keith got home that night he told me that at the recording session he would leave the room whenever he got so dizzy he wondered if he was making sense.

M a r c h 1

Last night I went out to dinner with my friends Ellen and Mary. Ellen said it was amazing that I haven't left Keith. She is the second person who has said that to me. I was too surprised to answer. I didn't know what to say. Leaving Keith has never occurred to me. I love him, he is my favorite. Besides, a person can't walk out on someone she loves when she is so desperately needed. Leaving Keith would kill him. I couldn't live with myself. It isn't an option.

What I hate is being in a position where I *can't* walk out. I hate his being sick and putting us in a position where we are no longer equal. If we were equal, then I could think about leaving, escaping. I don't think I ever would, but at least I could consider it; I would have an option. I hate this situation. But I can't leave Keith. It's never occurred to me not to see this through.

It's true that I am angry at Keith for being sick, but I can't take my anger out on him. Somehow, somewhere, I'll have to find a place for my anger, because I can't let it drive us apart.

My family is in trouble. The only way out is for the three of us to stay together. Otherwise whatever good there is left will be gone; we will have given way to the pressures.

March 3

Saturday night Mother took Luke to my parents' house in Brooklyn, and Keith and I went out to dinner. It felt good, so normal and healthy.

When Mother brought Luke home she left off an inspirational book by Rollo May with two notes inside, one a message from Dick with the name of a nursing service that comes to your home, the other a line from the Reverend Harcourt, a friend of my parents, saying that he knows what a difficult time this must be for everyone and that they pray for Keith every Sunday. The notes just made me angry. I hate Keith's being viewed as a terminal case, good intentions and realities aside.

The past few days I've been waking up nervous, with my teeth grinding. Sunday morning I woke up in tears, but I couldn't remember what I had dreamt. Felt selfish and mean as I kept thinking about the difference between not wanting Keith to have AIDS and not wanting to have a husband who has AIDS. Keith cheered me up a little by being loving and sweet.

We took the bus up to the Museum of Natural History. Good to be out as a family.

In the evening we put on a Michael Jackson record and watched Luke dance. Jumping around with Luke, we remembered how Keith and I would drink and dance to the same song three years ago. This was just as much fun—we all got the giggles—but so different. When Keith and I let our hair down now it is within the structure of our family—the two of us with Luke. When Keith and I are alone we are more subdued. We are getting more loving with each other, but Keith's responses to things seem new to me. I am not sure how to get on his wavelength the way I used to. The wavelength has changed.

Sometimes I feel that I am married to a man I hardly know. Believing in the marriage, loving the man, but not quite knowing who or what I'm dealing with.

At my last session with Susan she asked me about why I wasn't taking an active, enthusiastic role in resuming our sex life. We spoke about how I felt tainted by Keith's illness. Keith can tell I feel that way. He feels marked and shamed. Can't come to terms with the fact that his semen is poisonous to me. I can't either.

"Enthusiastic" seemed such an inappropriate word. I feel like a period of mourning should be observed before I think about resuming. Whatever kind of sex life we work out will be different, will have to be different than sex used to be. There are so many things to come to terms with. Keith looks different, he feels different. He looks sick. He feels bony and frail. I need to get used to his different body. And then there is the even bigger dilemma: we can touch, but how much? Sex used to imply abandon; now it must involve restraint. The limit seems to vary with everything we read, everyone we talk to. Kissing is fine, but not deep kissing. Some sources say intercourse is fine as long as the man wears a condom and withdraws, but other sources say intercourse even with a condom is risky. Doesn't anyone know for sure? Are we supposed to make our own decisions? A quagmire of questions and conflicting opinions that we feel ill-equipped to confront. We both are too emotionally frail.

I wonder if we will ever make love again. The thought that we won't terrifies me. Makes me feel something is dead when we are both working to prove that nothing will die. Keith has put packages of condoms in the bag that holds his drugs, but the sight of them is a complete turnoff. They seem part of a farce to me. Condoms are not enough. We both know that. A whole new way of physical love needs to be learned. I know that but I want to deny it. I cannot get used to this and most of me wants to prove it wrong. Our sex life seemed to overshadow so much before, put our problems in the background, made us feel powerful. Now that exists only in memory, and the memory makes the present worse. Sex can't conquer anything now. Sex has become the symbol of AIDS and the victim of AIDS. I feel completely defeated.

After all, sex is always scary. Under the best of circumstances the emotions it uncovers seem earth-shattering. This is going to take so much patience. Patience and faith. I must not give in to the frustration when it all seems hopeless. And so often it does. When I am in bed with Keith, longing for him, my defenses are down. And when my defenses are down I realize I want to scream and cry and have Keith take the pain away. But he can't. My need only exposes his pain. Sex has begun to seem like a Pandora's box that shouldn't be opened. We've worked out so much in the past few months, beginning to see a new way to be. The subject of sex just puts us back at square one. Makes us feel totally defeated. Instead of symbolizing our closeness, sex symbolizes the disease and our separateness. I reach out to Keith and feel nothing but anger and frustration.

Or I deny those feelings. Once I reached for Keith in the middle of the night and waited for him to say, Never mind, it's O.K., I will make love to you and all the past months will be proved wrong; it has all been a bad dream. Of course he couldn't respond. In the morning I was mortified at how irresponsible I was, at what an impossible position I had put Keith in. And I shudder when I remember Keith's pushing me away.

M a r c h 4

Woke myself up out of a nightmare. Luke and I were on a fire
escape above a burning building, I feeling certain that I was
losing my family in the fire. After the fire was out, I carried
Luke down the fire escape into the courtyard of the building to
try to find my family. I went up to a man who I thought was
my brother, Robert. The man looked identical to Robert but
said he didn't know me. I knew everyone was gone. Interesting
to me that the family I was concerned about losing was my
mother, father, and Robert, not Keith—he didn't play any part
in the dream or my thoughts. This was the first dream I've had
since Keith got sick that wasn't about Keith. Now that the
nightmare of November is less vivid to me I'm beginning to
focus more on myself, on my needs and fears. I must on some
level be worrying about whether my family will keep being
there for me. Will the stigma of Keith's illness alienate them?
There is so much unspoken in my family life these days—with
Keith as well as my parents—that I sometimes feel pervaded by
a vague sense of shame. That feeling of shame must be where
the insecurity about my family comes from.

M a r c h 5

Last night while Keith was in the bathroom I lay in bed and
cried. Warm, silent tears. I was thinking about London. Being
able to cry over that time at last felt good. I was finally acknowledging how horrible it had been. I hadn't allowed myself
to do that until now. It was a relief to admit to myself how
frightened and miserable I've been. It's true what Susan and Dr.
Michaels have been saying—it's better to let it out than try and
keep it in. Which makes me worry about Keith. Only a few
times since he's been home has he cried, admitted he was

frightened. It isn't in Keith's nature to give in to feelings of fear or self-pity. Keith is a fighter and he sees those emotions as signals of defeat. In many ways I admire his façade. But his emotions must be eating him up inside. I know he lies awake staring into the darkness. But I don't ask him what he is feeling. I'm scared to ask. It feels like too big a question. I tell myself that he'll tell me when he's ready.

After I cried I felt at peace. Finally I felt as though I could escape the particulars of my life long enough to get an overview.

Somewhere in the last six months there must have been turning points so subtle they've gone unnoticed. I can only think of different modes of feeling, not how I moved from one to the next. I remember London as panic and despair interspersed with moments of supernatural strength that seem to have come out of a vacuum. Coming home was confusion and fear. The weeks Keith was in St. Margaret's were exhaustion and anger, with a heavy dose of loving my son. When I think of what's been going on with us since Keith came home from St. Margaret's the picture gets more confused. From the days immediately after his return I remember only the routines—shoes off and hands washed whenever anyone entered the apartment, Clorox on the kitchen floor each night, meals prepared, Luke attended to. That was the period when I felt I worked as hard as I could each day and thanked God every night as Keith put Luke to bed. I didn't think, I didn't feel, we didn't really talk, and in memory everything is a total blur. That lasted through Christmas.

What's been happening in the last couple of months I'm not sure. Keith is getting physically stronger, and somehow I'm getting more confused. I know how to respond to a life-and-death crisis, but I don't know how to respond to the ongoing uncertainty of our lives. When I was holding Keith's hand and praying he'd make it through the night all my emotions were focused and clear. But now they're ambivalent, and I'm frightened to look at what lies beneath the surface. That's what Susan has been trying to get me to do, to look beneath the surface.

March 6

Keith's fever went up to 103.2 last night. We were both afraid that he would have to go back into the hospital, but Dr. Davis wasn't concerned. Keith slept through the night and woke up normal.

March 8

So exhausted. Yesterday morning Keith woke up with a slight fever but wouldn't cancel our appointment with Dr. Gorman or his afternoon business meeting. By late evening his fever had gone up to 104. I went into anxiety overdrive. Called Dr. Davis, who said to put Keith in a cold shower and keep giving him Tylenol. After the shower Keith got back in bed and I put cold compresses on his forehead. Turned off the lights and put on Mozart. Rubbed ice on his temples and tried to will his fever down. When he started drifting off to sleep, I called his brother, Michael, to make sure he would be available to watch Luke if Keith had to go to the emergency room (if his fever went over 104) during the night. Organized a sitter for the morning so I could take Keith to Dr. Davis.

Dr. Davis thinks Keith has the flu. He heard some pneumonia in Keith's left lung. He prescribed erythromycin and Septra just in case PCP is coming back. Gave Keith until Tuesday to get well. If Keith isn't better then he wants to put him in the hospital.

I worry a lot about Keith's pushing himself, not taking care. I suppose he is still learning about this disease—how much he can push himself, what happens if he does. It is obvious to me that a person with AIDS can never pretend he is well, never ignore any symptom of illness or hope it will go away.

I think Keith will get well on the antibiotics this time, but I feel that he is approaching a personal crisis. I think he is questioning who he is now that he has AIDS. He is fighting so many battles inside himself. I worry that they might kill him. It is so unfair that he spent all his life working out having had polio and now he has to figure out how to live with AIDS. The way he worked out living with polio isn't going to work now.

Keith and I have talked about leaving Dr. Gorman. At our last session Dr. Gorman talked about Keith's anger stopping his creativity. I think Keith feels that, since he has been denied a future, his dreams for the future must now be considered mere fantasies. Keith's daydreams used to nourish his creativity. It isn't anger that is stopping Keith's creativity: it is a lack of things to nurture it. Dr. Gorman also talked about turning what is perceived as oppression into recognition of your own power. It didn't really click. I agreed with part of what he said, that a sick person has a tremendous amount of power. But the power is limited to the realm of that person's personal relationships; Keith has tremendous power within our home. But what about the outside world? What has happened to his power there? Keith's position in the workings of the world is terribly important to him—and now his position fluctuates with his health.

Sometimes I think that our money would be better spent on a private therapist for Keith. Keith doesn't want to do that, but he also dislikes going to Dr. Gorman. He views the sessions as a pill he has to take: "You have AIDS, you should see a counselor." I feel that Dr. Gorman has been unable to come up with an inventive, individual, creative approach to this disease. He counsels as if he has a pamphlet on how to live with AIDS. He doesn't tune in to us enough as individuals.

And I'm not sure I agree with Dr. Gorman when he says that Keith is more in touch with his mortality than I am. I think that when someone first learns that he is seriously ill the desire to get well is so powerful that working to get strong becomes the main priority, not thinking about death. If the patient manages to recover, manages to feel relatively well again, does surviving PCP then seem much different from avoiding a falling brick on the street, when he looks back on it? Can a sick person really believe that he is going to die when he doesn't feel sick? I don't think so. I'm not saying that Keith hasn't thought a great deal about dying. I just think it's something he shuts out when he feels well—and maybe that's all to the good. Perhaps that way of coping should be encouraged. I have great faith in Keith's inventiveness in regard to his own life. While he is living his life I am not sure it does any good to think about dying.

Some of the things Dr. Gorman says offend me. It is all right for him to feed us the idea of infinite possibilities within a new given in our lives. That idea is O.K. But when he makes it sound like a commercial for Coke I think he is way off base. "You can have lots of fun with this disease, play jokes," he said. And then he laughs over an imagined scenario of a man with AIDS having dinner with friends, coming out of the kitchen and announcing to the dinner party, "The soup is great, I just tasted it," and the horrified looks of the other dinner guests. Silly, pointless, a waste of time, is what goes through my mind.

But I am resisting leaving Dr. Gorman because I'm scared of losing a time set aside for Keith and me to talk about AIDS. I'm afraid that we will never talk about it if we don't go down to his office every week. Sit in his tiny, depressing office with the broken radiator and electric heater and feel that everything that comes out of our mouths has to relate to the big A-I-D-S, which, when I am sitting in that tiny office, I imagine to be

84

stamped on a banner floating above our heads somewhere near the ceiling.

But that is precisely why we should leave, because everything that is said in that office is about AIDS. As if we are defined by being victims of AIDS, not people who had a life before AIDS, who want to continue living as complete human beings, who need to fit AIDS into our lives, not our lives into AIDS.

I would leave except that I still have the hope that if we keep going I'll eventually figure out how to get in bed with my husband and feel close to him. I don't want to live my life getting tense every time he enters the room. I want to talk about what is going on here, in this apartment. And I want to talk to Keith about it.

March 12

So sick of illness I could scream. Keith got better but then Luke got sick. He was miserable. Couldn't leave Luke with Keith because Keith was too weak to take care of him, and what energy he has is spent working on the music for a Tyson's food commercial he's recording this weekend. I couldn't take Luke out because he was sick and it's been so cold and wet outside. Luke was waking up every few hours at night and being clingy and weepy during the day. Saturday through Wednesday felt like one long day.

When Luke was born time changed. Exhaustion, confusion, and intimate elation blurred the difference between day and night. Everything melted together. The high point of the day might be 3 A.M., when I saw Luke staring at me, content and relaxed after he finished nursing. The low point might be 4 P.M., when I realized that the sun was going down and I hadn't had enough time to myself to wash my face or get out of my pajamas. I've been thinking about that time because I am as exhausted now as I was when Luke was a newborn. But when Luke was a newborn there was a sense of joyful purpose. Now there is only dread.

The responsibilities of being the only well person in the household are heavy. I have a lot of feeling "Who's going to help me?" and "Nobody understands how hard this is." Feeling sorry for myself. Want something to change—want money, want to be in the country, want help. I want more options, easier alternatives.

Last night I woke up crying in the middle of the night. I heard myself saying, "I don't want Keith to die." This time my tears didn't comfort me. I felt panicky. I don't want Keith to die— that feeling is as basic as breathing. To comfort myself I told myself I don't need to worry about that now. He is not dying now. This death fear isn't an intuition, I told myself. It can't be. I won't let myself think that way. Perhaps I am just now feeling the full weight of the panic I suppressed all last fall while Keith was so sick. I will myself to accept that as an explanation.

I am so tired of looking at life as a state that needs to be cherished, held on to, tentatively maintained—an interim state. I want to see life as the given, the foundation, not a fluke or borrowed time. I want to believe in the future. What I have to do now is decide that believing in the future is how I am going to live from now on. Living as if Keith is going to die seems impossible to me. Keith, Luke, and I are alive now and as long as we are alive we are alive forever. No more not making plans because they might be sabotaged by illness. The best way to live is with faith in the future. I think it is the way people are meant to live, even if they are dying. It must be nature's way, because it is the only way that feels right.

M a r c h   1 3

Had such a sad morning. Went to Susan and cried and cried. I was preoccupied and distracted before my session because I had dreamt that I had found a new man to marry—a man I didn't love but appreciated and enjoyed. At first I was horrified that I would dream such a thing, then realized that part of me is thinking about Keith dying and me living. When Keith dies it will hurt so much. But how long is he going to be sick? Will he die in two months or forty years?

I guess I'm coming to terms. With what I'm not sure. I want to say that I'm coming to terms with the fact that Keith will die, but my last journal entry was about believing we should live as if he isn't going to die. In fact, the last ten pages of this journal look like an exercise in ambivalence. I am optimistic then pessimistic; I reach out then retreat inward. Perhaps my ambivalence is what I need to make peace with.

When I got home in the early afternoon Luke was napping. Keith said he had written a flute part in the Tyson music. He got out the score, I got out my flute, and we played through it. I felt nothing but pleasure.

Later in the afternoon Luke walked up to Keith while Keith was writing a chart at the piano. Keith stopped what he was doing, put Luke on his lap, and sang and played in the outer octaves while Luke banged away at the keys in front of him. I looked at them and marveled at my talented husband and son. Then, this evening, Keith got in bed with a fever and I became angry at Luke because he wanted to eat his dinner on a tray in bed with his father (a very messy undertaking) instead of at the table.

March 15

Last night Keith woke up calling, "Betsy! Luke!" He said that he had had a nightmare in which I was off at a party and he was home alone. The phone rang and there was a crazy person speaking unintelligibly on the line. He said that he was afraid he was a burden to me.

Keith was shaking. I guessed that the crazy person on the line represented the feelings he has that he can't express. He was calling out to Luke and me to save him from his fears. He must feel guilty about the depth of his need for us. I told him that he wasn't a burden, that I wanted to care for him. Platitudes.

Today was the recording session for the Tyson job. I played the flute part. It felt great to be a professional musician again. It was like the days before Keith got sick—a wonderful respite from our roles as sick person and caretaker. At the recording studio in his role as producer and composer Keith was well. When Keith came home Luke got out of bed and danced to the tape—ooohing and aahing, clapping when it was over.

March 16

Luke didn't wake up until nine-thirty this morning. It felt as if we had slept until noon. Keith cooked breakfast. We all went to the Seminary Park. During nap time I went to the movies by myself. When I got home Keith and Luke and our home seemed warm and precious.

Last night Keith said that he gets scared. Said that he doesn't want to die because he has so much fun "here." That made me feel good. I need to know I am important to him now, that our life together gives him pleasure—it makes me feel that the present is worthwhile.

Keith also said that he was feeling "funny"—dizzy and cold. I suggested he talk to Dr. Davis about what to expect: How is he going to get sicker? How is he going to die? Can anyone say?

Keith said that he would like to die at home. Then he said that he didn't want to talk about dying anymore. He said he knows that he is repressing a lot, but that repression is part of the human condition. He said the thing to do now is to live in the present, since nobody knows what will happen anyway.

That may be easier for the sick person to say and do than the healthy person. For both of us it takes more bravery and courage than I ever imagined. Keith fears death, so living in the present helps to negate death. Sometimes I get jealous of him because he doesn't have to fear the future after he dies. I fear his dying and how it will feel after he is gone.

Each day I wake up like a child with a big worry—tense and angry. Then, as I enter the day, everything begins to seem all right. When the sun goes down the anxiety starts again. After Keith is asleep I get sad and lost. Last night I started crying while I was brushing my teeth. I wake up in the night and worry: What will I tell Luke if Keith gets sick again? How will I deal with Luke's anger and sadness when I am hurting? Should I make plans now concerning Keith's dying at home or going to the hospital? Am I jumping the gun? Will these things take care of themselves? Do we have years?

Keith started back on a regime of Tibetan medicine. They sent him two more pills, one for his liver and the other for his lymph glands.

* * *

Mother called Sunday to say that she wakes up in the middle of the night and thinks that I should be in a bank training program, or at least working. "What are you living on these days?"

"Should be working." What does she think I'm doing here? I've never worked harder in my life. I don't know how to explain to her that I can't leave my home now—can't leave it in the care of any other person. What does she think is going on here anyway?

At my last session Susan said that my feelings toward my mother were exacerbated because I have a need for her now: I want her support.

Sometimes I keep thinking it would get rid of some tension between my mother and me if I told her how Keith got sick. I just don't want to. I feel it is nobody's business. But there is also a strong part of me that wants to defend and explain my man.

Michael Callen called to ask Keith if he would be part of a musical AIDS benefit (the performers would be People with AIDS) he was planning. Keith said no. He said that he did not want to be part of anything that was part of dying, of doom. He felt that the celebration of talent was being used to accentuate the tragedy of AIDS and he doesn't want to have his life, or his talent, viewed as a tragedy. I understand Keith's point of view, and in some ways I admire it. But I shudder at his loneliness.

March 17

Today Keith had an appointment with Dr. Davis, who told him he is doing really well. Keith asked him how AIDS patients die. Dr. Davis said that each time a person with AIDS gets sick it is a crisis. He said that treatment is so much better than it used to be that he thinks survival rates for this year will be eighty percent. "Eighty percent surviving for how long?" I asked bitterly. "What is considered surviving?" The whole discussion made me angry. But I always feel some anger when Keith goes to the doctor. It reminds me that he is sick. And sometimes it makes me almost jealous of him: He's getting cared for, and I'm not.

My sister Rachel called to tell me she's pregnant. I said congratulations, how wonderful, when is the baby due? She was relieved at my reaction because she'd been afraid that I would be upset by her news, jealous. I told her that was silly; I'm glad for her. It wasn't until later that night that I realized I was imagining I was she, remembering when I was pregnant with Luke, my pride and pleasure in announcing it to my family.

March 18

A day of errands. Felt pissed off and tired. Ordered up a pizza for dinner and got drunk.

March 19

Keith is retiring and distant. More so than usual. It is as though he is retreating from the world. Retreating from me. Retreating into himself as if he has given up, lost his energy to fight. It makes me want to scream to see him calmly accepting his illness as his fate. Especially because I know inside he isn't really accepting it.

I took Luke to see the boats at the Twenty-third Street pier this morning. After supper I went to the movies across the street. When I got home Keith was lying in bed watching television. Didn't want to talk, said I was interrupting his program.

March 20

Black day. Tears and feeling desperate, powerless and alone. Looking at everything squarely and hating it all. Especially angry at Keith. Feel betrayed by him because he is pushing me away.

Keith went with Wayne to the movies. I have to admit it was nice having him out of the house.

March 21

I took Luke to the Whitney on the bus. We had a great time. Luke liked the big blue elevators best.

I told Keith that he has to talk to someone, that he was being distant and I felt shut out. I have no adult life with him, not to mention the frustrations of our sex life, or rather our lack of a sex life. I told him that I felt that he was taking good care of himself, and would continue to do so, but it seems to me that he feels he can only take care by shutting himself off from other people, i.e., me. Said there was no point in my hanging around if we don't have a life together.

Keith said that he didn't want to open old wounds, that the problems were old, and that if I continued hounding him he would get upset and then he would get sick. (How do you argue with *that?*)

In the morning Keith said I had made him so angry he couldn't sleep. I had slept great.

March 22

Keith felt fevery this evening. He said that he wanted to go to church tomorrow morning (Palm Sunday) and then out to brunch before his recording session at three. I said that it would be crazy to do so much—that he was being unrealistic, and that I wouldn't be able to enjoy myself, knowing that he was doing too much. Keith said he would never push himself too hard; we should wait until tomorrow, see how he felt, then make our plans. One more "wait and see." I lost my temper, said he was driving me crazy. Why didn't he move into a monastery, shut everyone else out, and just concentrate on taking care of himself in his own depressed way? He said I was making everything worse. Said he was worried about money, that all his friends remind him of the past, that he can't get used to condoms, and what was I upset about?—he's handling everything great. I was the one making these problems insurmountable, starting arguments. I keep thinking that people get divorced for less.

We went to church the next morning, but had lunch at home.

March 24

Keith went on the bus with Luke and me to the Abingdon Square playground. Luke was thrilled to have his Daddy with us. At home during lunch Keith said, "I wonder how I can find a psychiatrist?" It shouldn't be a competition, but I feel that I've scored a minor victory. Maybe more over my powerless self than over Keith.

March 25

Susan recommended a therapist for Keith. I'm hoping that the strings that tie our marriage together will stop strangling it at last.

March 27

Keith went to church this evening. My friend Karen came over while he was gone. A wonderful antidote for my feeling shabby and at odds with life—she gave the impression that she thought that our life was cozy and rich. Luke thought she was wonderful and asked her to dance. I love my women friends.

COMING INTO SPRING

March 29

Keith and I went to evening mass. The Easter story is almost too much to hear after this awful winter. Something moved inside me which was way beyond tears or sentimentality.

March 31

I loved Easter morning. Luke was thrilled to wake up to his Easter basket, and he caught right on to the idea of an Easter-egg hunt. Keith gave me a beautiful long, white summer nightgown. We went uptown and walked across Central Park, Luke chasing his orange ball.

April 2

Two magically beautiful days—sunny, clear, and warm. Luke has spring fever and is refusing to take his nap. We've been going to Abingdon Square in the morning, the Seminary Park in the afternoon. Sat on the park bench yesterday morning thinking that there is no place I would rather be.

April 4

I find myself dissolving into dizzying confusion when Keith enters the room—emotional paralysis from feeling such intense love and attraction combined with so much anger. In therapy I find myself talking in the bleakest terms about Keith and me, and I suppose about my life in general. Do I really feel as angry, cheated, powerless, and abused by Keith and our life as I sound? I come home and have a hard time believing what I just said.

Susan is very supportive of my anger and the dark side of my emotions. I think she is trying to get me to confront things in my relationship with Keith that I never thought about before, after which I will be able to feel that I am acting independently, with my eyes open, seeing my choice as my own—not a choice made in rebellion against my parents, or out of a need to nurture someone weaker than myself.

The thing I am most afraid of is feeling that I have no choices—and then feeling bitter as a result.

Spring fever. Waking up at 5 A.M., very hyper but not thinking very clearly.

April 7

Keith found a used-car ad in the paper. We went down to Tribeca, saw a twelve-year-old SAAB, and bought it. I am having such lovely fantasies of the three of us adventuring this summer.

Got home to a message on the machine from Calvin Klein asking Keith to write the music for his spring fashion show. Life seems promising again. Amazing what the promise of money can do. Actually, it's not just the money—it's the feeling of having a life again, with Keith working and plans and fantasies about the future. Things to look forward to.

April 11

Fighting off some kind of flu today. Couldn't get anything together. By late afternoon told Keith that I had to lie down. Went into the bedroom while Keith got Luke his supper. Felt Keith resented my being sick. Felt he couldn't/wouldn't give me any sympathy. He said he was afraid that he was going to catch my illness. My interpretation was that he didn't want me to be sick because then I couldn't care for him and Luke.

I felt sorry for myself. Lying alone in the bedroom I started to think about my room when I was growing up. I remembered getting dressed in that room and looking in the mirror, knowing that, whether I was happy with my life at that moment or not, I could always wrap my arms around myself and feel that the boundaries of my world were enclosed within that semicircle. I was self-sufficient and self-contained. What the hell happened to that feeling? Why can't I lie down by myself even when I'm sick without feeling that I'm failing my family? Have I no identity but wife to Keith, mother to Luke, caretaker to both?

April 16

Today I took Luke up to visit Keith in the loft where he's working (he shares time there with four other musicians). It's in a building that is exclusively rehearsal lofts and is quite a scene—black walls covered with graffiti and characters wandering around who make MTV look tame. Luke was fascinated. We found Keith sitting at his synthesizer. He put Luke on his lap and let him experiment with the sounds it made. Then he said to me: "I want to play you what I've written. It's so beautiful. It's all about you." Keith's eyes were glowing. He sang: "You gave me hope, you gave me life, you gave me a chance to be myself, you gave me love, you gave me life. . . . You gave me strength when I was down, you gave me shelter from the world, you gave me love, you gave me life."

I sat on the floor with Luke in my lap. I had forgotten that Keith could always say with his music what he had difficulty saying face to face. I had forgotten that. I swore I'd never forget it again. And I felt like crying. I felt like crying because a tension had relaxed. Tension from a fear I hadn't even admitted to myself until I heard Keith playing—the fear that I might never again hear Keith, with his eyes shining and a grin of pride on his face, play a new song for me. And here he was singing about the last eight months of our life with love and appreciation for me. Giving me his interpretation of the struggle. An interpretation remarkable for its absence of pain, anger, guilt, or shame.

When he stopped singing I couldn't say anything—nothing was appropriate. I looked at him and smiled. We smiled at each other. I felt complete unto ourselves again, as I had not done for a very long time. I realized that's what I've been missing most—the joy we used to have in being alone together, in sharing ourselves with each other. It made me think of our time in Denver.

Denver. Thirteen years ago. I remember one afternoon coming home from the supermarket carrying bags of groceries. It was the summer before we were married. I opened the gate to the backyard and walked up the stairs to the door of our apartment, the top floor of a two-story, two-family house. I remember standing in the middle of the stairs and looking down at the garden Keith and I had planted in the yard and thinking, "I am completely happy. I will never be this happy again." I wasn't right. I thought that again after Luke was born, but something in me knew enough to look around and take stock. Value this.

We had left England in February or March. Keith wanted to continue his career and felt he needed a more secure base to continue his creative life. I wanted to go home, face my family, and leave them again with a true plan, a true leaving. I needed to tell them I was going to live my life with Keith. (That's what had happened in London. We came to know that we always wanted to live together.)

I went back to my parents' house in Brooklyn Heights. Keith stayed with friends a few blocks away. We were planning to get jobs and save enough money to rent an apartment.

The day that Keith went to get his picture taken for his hack license, however, he had a terrible headache. Then a fever. Then a rash. The doctor diagnosed a case of mononucleosis and hepatitis. He left the friends he was staying with and moved in with his parents on Long Island. I got a job as a salesgirl in a store on Lexington Avenue. On my days off I drove my parents' car out to Long Island to see Keith. It took him about a month to get well enough to even begin to think straight about the future.

His cousin, a guitarist in Denver, called Keith to say that his band needed a piano player. Was Keith interested? As soon as Keith was well enough to travel he left for Denver. I stayed at my parents' for another month, until I had enough money to pay for my plane ticket and a little extra to set up some sort of life in Denver.

We bought a ten-year-old white Cadillac from an old man, fins and all, for $250. That Cadillac became what some people's country houses are to them, our second home. We unwound in it. In the middle of the night we would go driving around town. Case the deserted streets. Plan our future. Look at houses and say, "I could live there, but I'd rather live . . ."

I took a job in a restaurant four mornings a week (eleven to two—it was morning to us). Keith played in his cousin's band in Holiday Inns and honky-tonk bars. ("If you hear gunshots," his cousin had told him, "keep playing. They never shoot at the band while they're playing.") He came home from work at two or three in the morning.

We used to eat a meal around six, before Keith left for work. In the afternoon I would go outside to our garden and pick some vegetables. Keith's piano was in our kitchen. While I cooked dinner he would sit at the piano and sing and play. After we had eaten and Keith had left for work I would clean up our dinner things and get out my flute, and play until 1 or 2 A.M. I loved breaking the silence of the hours in the middle of the night with my flute playing. And I loved the silence between 2 and 3 A.M. when I would wait for Keith to come home.

Our first winter in Denver there was more snow than I had ever seen in my life. All through the winter months the sound of traffic outside was muffled by the packed snow.

We were both young enough to feel that time was infinite. That the future was limitless. That nothing was irreparable. That we could achieve all we wanted. But we weren't frivolous. To both of us our life together was something wonderfully serious and significant. I have in my closet the notebooks we would leave on the kitchen table (a picnic table we stole from the backyard when we moved in) for writing notes to each other. We took such care in communicating.

I remember one Thanksgiving. We sat down together with ceremony. After dinner we walked around our neighborhood, came home, and made love. Later that evening we played the Mozart *Flute Concerto in G* together, Keith playing the orchestral part on the piano.

We lived in Denver almost four years. We changed a lot in that time. We decided to get married. I decided to go to music school. Keith became frustrated with his cousin's band and quit. He got a commission from a local church to write a rock mass. It was a success: Keith was interviewed by the Denver papers, we went to dinner with patrons of the Denver Symphony. Keith was commissioned to write a piece for the Denver planetarium—a forty-minute show under the "stars" with a live orchestra and singers in honor of the fleeting and dim comet Kohoutek. He wrote a score for an ABC Afternoon Special. We moved into a larger apartment.

I was devoted to my flute teacher and did a lot of playing and teaching myself. Keith got a grant to write a score for a new musical by Mary Chase that was scheduled to open the Denver Center for the Performing Arts. I was ready to stay forever.

Keith wasn't. His musical project with Mary Chase was canceled because of a lawsuit with the actors' union. Money became tight again. Keith was disgusted with the musical life in Denver. He got a job playing in Montreal and thought he would visit New York before he came home.

I remember Keith coming home from New York. He walked into our apartment and said that he hated it. Denver was the middle of nowhere, exciting things were happening in New York, and if they weren't always exciting at least they were professional.

I hated hearing that. I liked our life in Denver.

But I was twenty-one and Keith was twenty-eight. Different

things were important to us. Keith had outgrown Denver. He needed to be part of a bigger world. When he came back from his trip to New York he said that he had to move back there, and if I didn't want to go with him he was going to go alone.

So Keith went alone. I guess it was out of spite that I stayed. I was angry that he was ending what I wanted to continue.

I gave in and went to New York about six weeks after Keith had left. We moved into a tiny walkup on the Upper West Side. We fought all the time—over morning coffee, on the subway, up and down the stairs to our apartment.

We had no money. We used to buy our groceries at Zabar's because they took MasterCharge and we could charge our milk and eggs and bread. We walked because we couldn't afford the bus. I had a job I hated as a receptionist. Keith was accompanying a cabaret singer at night. We wouldn't see each other for days. It was really better that we didn't. I was furious at him for choosing this over our life in Denver.

Eventually we went to see a psychiatrist whom Keith had gone to while he was in music school and got some counseling. Our fights got fewer.

We moved into our present apartment on Twenty-third Street and Eighth Avenue. I remember signing the lease and then sitting in a coffeeshop listing what possessions we could sell to pay the rent. I started at NYU. Keith started teaching. I got some flute students. Keith got fairly regular accompanying work. We settled in.

Our life grew. Keith was working steadily. He got some freelance work doing arrangements for *Saturday Night Live.* He started writing music again. He could afford to perform with his own band. I taught and studied. Waitressed on the weekends. We were struggling but it all seemed to be going forward.

Those years are hard to think about now. I miss them desperately. I miss the way we built our life and then used it, built just enough security so that we could bounce off it. Getting just enough money in the bank so that Keith could make a demo, I could give a recital. Staying out till dawn, talking through the night. I remember practicing in the mornings on three hours of sleep and pots of coffee. Playing for Keith. Keith playing for me.

And then Luke was born, nine years after we moved back to New York. The year after Luke was born was a little like Denver, something felt the same. It is the feeling I've been missing until now, the feeling I wasn't sure if I'd ever have again—the feeling that we are complete unto ourselves, Keith, Luke, and I. How important Keith and I believed ourselves to be, immortal really. We were going to live forever and we were going to be better than the rest. Because this was better than the rest. Remembering that now breaks my heart. All I can think of is how innocent we were, how young.

April 26

I've lost my center. Completely. It happened two days ago when I went to have my blood tested. Dr. Davis had been telling Keith that it should be done, and he really put the pressure on during Keith's last appointment. He said testing me was the sane, responsible thing to do. He pointed out that a doctor couldn't treat me, care for me, in an intelligent manner without knowing if I am antibody positive or negative.

I felt bulldozed into having the test. If I'm positive I don't want to know. Why know now? That's what I've been telling myself—what good would knowing now do? I'm feeling healthy. But then Dr. Davis brought up Luke. If I'm positive, Luke could be positive. It all sounds surreal, the making of a nightmare. I want to continue denying the possibility of the nightmare. But at the mention of Luke I felt that I had to face facts, and get it over with.

I remembered taking Luke for his checkup last December. Keith was in St. Margaret's then. I told Luke's pediatrician that Keith had AIDS. I remember feeling encased in anxiety—horrified by the implications of that statement. "Let's take this one step at a time," he had said. "There is no point jumping to conclusions until you are tested."

Keith says it's no big deal; he knows I'm negative. I can't tell if it's intuition telling him I'm negative or dread. He would feel so guilty if I were positive that he has convinced himself I'm negative. Either way he's no comfort. He's working all the time now.

Keith offered to come with me. So did my mother. Their offers of support didn't take away my feeling that I'm on my own with this dilemma. I decided I wanted to go by myself. I was determined to be strong, or rather, pretend to be. If I went alone I could pretend it wasn't such a major event.

The morning of my appointment I felt I was in a dream. Walked into Dr. Davis's office and realized how nervous and scared I was. Broke out in a rash on my chest. Dr. Davis gave me a physical, and when he listened to my heart he said it was racing so fast he couldn't tell what was going on.

Keith said that Dr. Davis had told him I was probably negative. When I was sitting in his office I could tell that he—and I—knew that there was a good chance I was positive. Talking to him brought back all the memories of doctors being serious with me in England.

All in all an incredibly alienating experience. Went to the lab room to have my blood drawn and the technician said, "I've never seen a woman in here." I wanted to say, "Thanks for letting me know how anomalous my situation is." But I couldn't even muster the energy for sarcasm.

Tears on and off the rest of the day. Does Keith know, does anyone know, what a positive result will mean to me? I'll feel that God has taken away from me all the things that I love, all my dreams, all the things I hope for, work for. Crying for myself, for Luke, for my unborn babies. I can't share my fears with Keith because I am so angry at him for putting me through one more emotional ordeal. And he feels guilty enough already. I'm terrified of how much I will hate Keith if I am positive.

Keith and I wouldn't be able to face each other if I am positive. It would be the end of us. And there would be the chance Luke was positive, that our baby could die.

April 30

This waiting is too hard. I've marked on the calendar when three weeks will be up, and worked out a plan in my mind so I can get through them. Decided to call Dr. Davis and tell him I would come in to review the results of my blood work, as planned, but I must not know the results of the AIDS test. I am going to call him and tell him to put on his best poker face and not let me guess at the answer. Tell him he has to do this because I can't handle a positive result. I couldn't care for Luke or Keith if the results are positive.

I know this is crazy. I won't call him.

My friend Karen came over Saturday night and said that I was torturing myself unnecessarily. That it will be all right, whatever happens.

May 5

So exhausted I've lost all perspective. Thursday afternoon Keith had an open-ended studio session to record the Calvin Klein music. That night I woke at 3:30 A.M. and he wasn't home. I panicked—sure he was killing himself working so late. I told myself he would have called if anything was wrong. Finally got back to sleep, the bed falling through the center of the earth. I dreamt of Rachel in my maternity clothes. I dreamt of myself tired and haggard meeting a well-dressed, successful-looking couple. The woman of the couple said that she was the man's partner. That every successful man needed a partner.

Friday was a daze. Keith slept all day. I kept Luke away so he could sleep.

Getting ready for bed Friday night Keith talked about the music he was writing. He said that he kept thinking he was writing the music for his funeral. I couldn't sleep.

Saturday Luke and I went to visit Keith in the studio. Luke sat in a chair at the board next to Keith playing with the controls (the unconnected ones). Kept saying, "More song, more song." Eating Keith's takeout breakfast. So proud he was sitting next to his Daddy at work, holding his own. Bopping to the music.

When Luke and I got home there was a message on the phone machine from Dr. Davis saying that the preliminary results of my blood work showed my blood to be normal. Helped a little.

Keith was home Sunday and we fought all morning. I was angry that I had worked so hard holding down the fort and now Keith finally had a day off and he was tense and exhausted. But that isn't really what's wrong. It's this sense of fear, terror really, always under the surface. I'm constantly bursting into tears.

Worrying and feeling impotent. It all seems so crazy. Keith writing this beautiful music, working suicide sessions in the studio, me at home taping a television program on experimental AIDS drugs.

I feel that everything important is out of my control.

Had a huge martini yesterday evening and danced around with Luke. The connection that numbs and heals.

May 9

I feel that I have cried and screamed myself out. Now I feel
that in imagining a positive result I have done so much crying
that I might as well get the results and finish out the anger and
despair. The reality of a positive test can't be much worse than
what I've been putting myself through.

Tuesday was the Calvin Klein fashion show. The whole event
seemed bizarre. I couldn't put AIDS out of my mind. Last year
the models and clothes looked beautiful to me. This year the
models looked anorexic. The whole event seemed like a bizarre
ritual: skeletal women parading down the runway, Keith's music in the background with lyrics about a life-and-death crisis,
which had no place in this celebration of artifice. None of it
made any sense. What did this have to do with our lives other
than the fact that Keith had made a lot of money from it? I
think Keith felt the same way. He had been upset because they
weren't using his music in the middle of the show. The politics
of working—his ego, their egos—had really gotten to him this
time. But we went out to lunch between shows and joked about
it all. With our newfound perspective we were comrades, and
we enjoyed that bond. The terror of waiting for my test lifted.
We relaxed together.

May 13

Sunday was Luke's second birthday. And Mother's Day. A light,
magical day. The apartment looked festive, airy, and flower-
filled. Luke was adorable—charming and proud. We had a small
party and celebrated at home. After the cake, Luke and his
friend Emma got in the bath together to play with their "deep-
sea divers," party favors that Keith had bought. Luke's friend
Jacob walked around in his diaper. Marianne, Donna-Maria,

and I (the mothers) drank champagne and toasted ourselves. In the late afternoon when the guests had gone, I felt content and happy. Having more babies no longer seemed important. I suppose it's been a symbol this past year. There are other ways to fill your house with children.

That evening Keith gave me a beautiful watch. It is perfect. I didn't care whether or not we could afford it. I deserved it.

The next day, Monday, Keith went for his appointment with Dr. Davis. As soon as Keith came home he reported that Dr. Davis had told him my test was negative. I felt blessed and lucky—as if a hundred pounds had been lifted from my shoulders. I enjoyed calling my family and telling them the news. I was touched by their relief, the strength of which gave away their previous concern. As I was getting ready for bed it occurred to me that now that I am officially well the imbalance in our marriage is even greater, although nothing has changed.

M a y 1 4

Keith announced that tomorrow night we are going to the Fashion Video Awards at the Palladium. I felt taken for granted. I wanted to be asked, not told. We had a terrible fight.

I felt bad afterward. Keith had made the announcement with such pride and excitement. Two of the commericals he worked on are up for awards that night, and I'm sure he was surprised and hurt that I wasn't as excited as he was. But I was worried that the night would be too much for him. He looked at me as if I were crazy when I expressed my concern—what had happened to my priorities? It's true that I used to be a lot more adept at juggling them.

Soon after Luke was born we were invited to Cornelia Guest's birthday party at Regine's. I was hesitant about leaving Luke with a sitter—I was still nursing him every few hours. So we hired a limousine and took Luke with us, as well as my brother and his girlfriend as the babysitters. Luke made an appearance at the party, then retired to his temporary nursery in the back of the car, watched over by Robert and Annie, who had the limo's bar and television to keep them entertained. When Luke woke up hungry, Annie brought me back to the limo and I nursed him.

I thought of that night and realized that I've lost the power of my inventiveness.

It's been too hard a month. I want to lick my wounds and recharge my batteries in my own way. Desperately trying to pull the center of gravity back from Keith and Luke toward myself.

I called the GMHC about a support group for caregivers of people with AIDS. They gave me the number of the woman who would know what group would be best for me. I called but she's out of town for a week.

May 20

We went to the Fashion Video Awards and had a very good time for a while. But the awards went on for hours. Afterward we went out to dinner because Keith couldn't bear to give in to his exhaustion. But we had to leave as soon as our food arrived—he suddenly felt faint and dizzy. The sight of food made him sick.

He was fine the next morning. In fact, Keith seems to have survived the last couple of weeks really well. I think going to his therapist is helping him enormously.

I'm feeling hungover from a weekend of family. My sister Ann came to town with her husband and children for a cousin's wedding. The wedding brought up the old appeal of security—everything being done as it "should be." Made me lose some pride and strength, made my life seem so very fragile compared to all those well-ordered lives. And, since the WASP ethos is built on the concept of getting your just deserts, I keep thinking: What did I do to deserve this? Did I do something wrong?

May 23

I took Luke to Abingdon Square this morning. While he played in the sand with another little boy his age, I sat on the edge of the sandpit chatting with the boy's mother. They live near Washington Square but walk the extra distance to Abingdon Square because of the drug users in Washington Square. "You never know," she said, "some of those children's parents could have AIDS."

May 28

We've finally decided to move. We'd talked about it before Keith got sick, but only now have we felt secure enough to be a bit adventurous again. I'm back to feeling that we are a self-contained family unit. Wherever we go will be home so long as Keith and Luke are with me.

Keith, Luke, and I drove Luke's friend Jacob and his mother, Marianne, down to the Market Square playground. It was sunny and green. Two men walked by, one leaning on the other. One looked healthy and strong and one very, very sickly, with KS lesions on his face. Looking at them I felt nauseous and weak in the knees. It made me count my blessings and made my heart break all at the same time. Marianne said, "That man has AIDS." Keith and I were silent. It was horrifying in the middle of all the children and green grass.

* * *

I went to the GMHC's support group for caregivers of PWAs for the first time. I was extremely nervous: Who are these people going to be? What will I get out of this?

The answer to the first question is that they are a group as varied as the population of New York, from a college professor with four grown children to a bartender in a well-known gay bar. I don't know the answer to the second question, but I'm committed to giving the group a try.

I was thunderstruck to see what a cross-section of society has been hit by AIDS. Lying awake that night I thought about all the members of my group and pictured each of us home with our loved ones, home with the ones we can't bear to lose, home praying in secret. I became enraged. I looked at Keith differently that night. I saw him as the victim of a huge injustice, an injustice not only of nature and fate, but also of society. What are you doing to him? I felt like shrieking. Why are you making him feel that he is wearing a scarlet letter on his chest? Why aren't you helping him?

May 29

Looked at two apartments, neither of them right for us. When we got home I became terrified. How can we make any changes? What if Keith gets sick? Where would our familiar things be?

Keith and I have decided that we must make a commitment toward the future or we will lose our minds. This is taking all my courage, especially in the evening. Then I feel that my future is frozen and if I step out on the ice it will crack.

We went to my cousin Max's house in Germantown for the weekend. We got the house in exchange for feeding his chickens. We arrived Friday afternoon. The SAAB started overheating on the Taconic and we only made it because we found a wonderful mechanic in Rhinebeck. Luke had a ball feeding the chickens and the cats and playing with Max's daughter's toys. I worried. I worried about Keith's health around all the animals, insects, and dust. I worried he would get sick and the car wouldn't start to take us home. God knows what would happen to him in the Rhinebeck hospital. At night when Keith and Luke were asleep, I wondered what we were doing—a sick man, a two-year-old, and I—in the middle of the countryside surrounded by chickens with a car that's unreliable at best.

June 3

Saturday we began to relax. In the evening we drove into Germantown to pick up some groceries and the newspaper. There it was on the front page: Perry Ellis dead of viral encephalitis. My stomach turned over and Keith turned white. I knew what Keith was thinking. I was thinking the same thing: If a millionaire can't be treated, what chance does Keith have?

Sunday was unusually hot, like an August day. We went to visit Virginia and Eric at their country house nearby and had a really nice time. Got away from feeling isolated and jinxed. That night the temperature dropped and a wind came up and it was heaven putting Luke to sleep in his room under an open window. Woke up feeling that the trip had worked. We were enjoying life again.

Monday morning we started the drive down. The SAAB started to overheat after about an hour. We stopped to get something to eat and let it cool down. Keith said he was feeling sick. We made it to a garage in Yonkers. The car wouldn't go over twenty m.p.h. and Keith was getting whiter and whiter. The mechanic at the garage said we could make it home—but the car died on the West Side Highway, at 120th Street. When I said we needed a taxi, Luke put out his hand and said, "Taxi," and one came along and stopped. Magic. Went to Virginia and Eric's Manhattan apartment on 110th Street, where Virginia put Keith to bed and sent her son to take care of the car and our belongings. Home and settled by nine. Trying to forget the feeling of panic on the West Side Highway. So scared and so very, very alone. Desperately wanted someone to take care of me, tell me what to do.

We are all recovering today.

June 1 6

Yesterday was Father's Day. Luke helped me make pancakes for his daddy. Then I gave Keith a shirt, and Luke gave him a picture he had drawn. Blue, brown, purple, pink, and yellow lines shooting across the page. Keith and I decided Luke is brilliant: the colors are Keith's colors exactly.

June 2 1

Took out a loan and have bought a new car. A car is a necessity—it is Keith's mobility now. Keith is working on getting his handicapped plates and parking permit.

We have named it Champagne Car. When we were looking over colors in the Honda brochure Keith said, "Champagne beige it is." Luke said, "Champagne car." The name stuck.

Keith loves his car. I consider it his because it is not only his mobility but also his second home. An extra sweater in the back, Tylenol and music tapes in the glove compartment. I think he feels safe in his car, as if he's in his own world, where nothing can harm him.

Yesterday Keith took Luke to the car wash. When they got home Keith and Luke played car wash in the kitchen sink. For an hour they washed and polished Luke's little plastic cars. To get the atmosphere right Keith put disco music on the radio.

SUMMER

D r. Davis has been talking on and off for weeks about Keith's starting on a new drug, ribavirin. Has said it is Keith's "insurance plan against dying." Says it kills the protein covering of the HIV virus. I don't really understand, but he said something to the effect that it doesn't kill the HIV virus, but stops it from attacking the white cells—stops it from being aggressive, or rather progressive. This is the second part of Dr. Davis's grand plan. He wants first to boost Keith's immune system with naltrexone, then stop the progression of the HIV virus with ribavirin.

Ribavirin hasn't been approved by the Food and Drug Administration. Dr. Davis mentioned about a month ago that we should consider flying to Mexico to get some. In Mexico ribavirin is an over-the-counter drug. Dr. Davis said that ribavirin is so expensive in the United States that it would be cheaper to fly to Tijuana, fill up a suitcase, and fly home than to try to get some here.

Now Dr. Davis says that it isn't safe to do that. The United States is cracking down on bringing drugs into the country. He has some in his office. Keith and I have figured it will cost about $100 a week. We don't have the money.

I wrote a letter to Keith's parents and his uncle asking for their help. I'm very proud of the letter. I think it's eloquent and tactful.

Going to my group has made it easier for me to ask for help. In fact, it has made me want to demand it.

Keith was hesitant to ask his family for help. He was evasive when I asked him why. Is it because he can't stand telling them he needs their help? Is he scared they will say no? I told Keith that they should be asked before we ask my family or our friends. It's right to do it that way. I said to Keith the same thing I wrote in the letter: that I'm sure as Keith's family they would want to know our situation.

July 8

Keith started ribavirin five days ago. It turned him into a madman. Nervous and hyper. Really manic. Hardly sleeping. Itching all over. He went to Dr. Davis and said he was jumping out of his skin. Said he was only sleeping three hours a night. Dr. Davis said he was doing great—when most people start on ribavirin they can't sleep at all.

Dr. Davis is cutting back the dosage.

No one has responded to my letters. I called Keith's dad. He said that he doesn't have the money, that he is living on a fixed income, that Keith's mother has been sick. Keith is so hurt.

Keith told Dick about his parents' not helping out. Dick said he was asking the wrong people. He is giving us the money.

July 10

Last night Luke woke up crying. I went in, changed his diaper, and sat in the rocker by his crib. When he had gone back to sleep I returned to bed. As I was drifting off he cried out for Mama. I went and sat by his crib again. He fell asleep at 4 A.M. I had been up for an hour. I felt claustrophobic and tense. Felt like making coffee and lying on the couch reading, but knew if I did I'd never make it through the day. So I went back to bed and stared at the ceiling. Then I fell asleep and dreamt about the past year.

I dreamt that we were all at home and it was just before dawn. Luke and I were going to go exploring. We found a door in the back of the hall closet, behind the coats. It went to a hallway. Off the hallway there were two sunny rooms with lots of nooks and crannies. I was excited. "I had forgotten we had this space," I said to myself. "It is our past." The rooms' closets were filled with the shampoos and deodorants and hairbrushes that we used to use in Denver. The discovery made me feel rich and satisfied. Carrying Luke, I continued exploring.

The hallway went on, but the rooms off it became more and more public. We passed a dining room set for dinner, but it was the dining room of a law office, set up for a conference meal. We walked through offices and public restrooms. We were walking through hotels. We stopped for coffee in a hotel-lobby coffeeshop and I began to want to find our way home.

I asked for directions and a man showed me a map. I couldn't remember the name of the building we lived in but I did remember what direction home was in. I carried Luke downstairs to get on a subway. Everything became alien and strange. Luke went limp in my arms. It was as if he were sleeping, but he had become weightless. When we got off the subway we were in another lobby. It was a hospital. I showed Luke's limp body to the doctors and they said that he was dead. My legs gave out—I collapsed in grief. I felt pure hatred projecting from my eyes.

The doctors started cutting his body into strips to analyze his illness. They gave me the fragments to take home. I went home with them, full of guilt because I had let him die, but when I got home Keith wasn't upset. He wasn't really anything. The grief and horror were all in me. I put Luke's head in a fishbowl to try to nurture it back to life. An eyeball moved. "If they hadn't cut you up you would be alive, I know you would be alive." Time stopped. Then Keith and I heard Luke laughing and shouting in the next room. Luke was alive in our house, and we had hidden rooms that were mine behind the hall closet. I had my rooms. And my past.

J u l y   1 2

Sometimes Keith talks about going away on a vacation. A vacation in the sun. Far away. But how can we go? Dr. Davis says that the sun is bad for people with AIDS—depletes the white blood cells or something. Keith used to love to bake in the sun. Now he wears long-sleeved shirts.

Keith and I don't say it to each other, but we are scared to go away, as if right here is all we trust to support us. I suppose in a way we view the rest of the world as hostile. It is a feeling I don't want to give in to. But reading the newspaper often feeds that feeling—reading about countries not letting people with AIDS in, testing immigrants' blood, not to mention articles on quarantining them. Keith and I joke about the articles in the paper, but I know they hurt him. They certainly upset me.

July 15

Can't sleep these days. I wake up at 2 A.M. feeling that this household is being pulled into a black hole of space, a vacuum of indecision, anger, and fear. It seems we've slowed down to a snail's pace—the weight of Keith's and my fears is too heavy for us to move forward. Our indecisions are freezing us. And the irony is that nothing is terribly wrong at the moment—the worst thing happening is that we are frustrated and bored.

I wonder if my going to my support group is enlarging the gulf between me and Keith. He tells me he thinks it is morbid, going somewhere just to talk about AIDS. I am enjoying the camaraderie of my group. I tell him we don't talk about AIDS, we talk about ourselves. My group meets on Tuesday evenings. Evening is a bad time to go out. Luke needs his bath and supper and Keith is at his lowest, often fighting a fever. Before I leave he moans about how sick he feels. I feel extremely guilty but know that I'd be so angry if I didn't go that I'd be no help to anyone at home. So I leave, and when I come home what I usually find is Luke (bathed and pajamaed) in bed with Keith watching TV, two dinner trays fixed by Keith (pizza is the preferred specialty) lying at the foot of the bed. Cozy and smiling.

Sometimes I feel like an intruder between Keith and Luke. A carrier of gloom and doom. Except for when he is feeling very ill or loses his temper, Keith is always optimistic and cheerful around Luke. During periods like these, when Keith and I are skirting the issues and avoiding our worries, I feel like a pall on their happiness. I suppose I am jealous of Keith putting on his best for Luke, while I feel I get his worst.

We don't have a buyer for our apartment. We can't find a place we really want to live in. Whatever we find that is possible we discard because we don't trust our judgment at this time. We're afraid. We say it doesn't matter that we haven't decided on a new space because we haven't sold our apartment yet—back to square one.

We have gone on some small adventures. Luke is giving us momentum. We went to the aquarium at Coney Island and walked on the boardwalk. We took the Staten Island Ferry one very hot evening and saw the Statue of Liberty. We drove back over the Verrazano Bridge with the sunroof open.

July 21

This morning Keith went to see Dr. Davis about the sores in his mouth. Dr. Davis said that they looked like herpes. They have been very painful and debilitating for about five days now. I am terrible with this kind of health problem when it comes to sympathy for Keith—I seem to have no patience. He is uncomfortable enough to be miserable but it isn't a serious enough problem for me to switch into my Florence Nightingale role. Hearing Keith moan about his mouth reminds me that he is sick and that this disease isn't going away. He is too uncomfortable for me to leave Luke with him for any length of time. Lots of feelings of being trapped and I hate them.

Constantly worrying about Keith. He is so white and thin. He went off ribavirin two weeks ago because he couldn't tolerate it. He is starting a lesser dose tomorrow. The plan is two weeks on, two weeks off. I don't understand how it can be good for him if it takes away his appetite and keeps him from sleeping.

Keith is on so many drugs. Or on and off them. If they don't have to be kept in the refrigerator, Keith keeps them in a plastic cosmetics bag. Diphenhydramine, naltrexone, tetracycline, metronidazole, lidocaine, folic acid, dapsone, Zovirax, triamcinolone cream, Mycelex.

Timelessness. Marooned in the present. No way of planning for the future. Like living in a vacuum. I feel it is killing us. Hot and sticky outside. Uncomfortable inside: Keith says air conditioning makes him cough and his skin itch. In any case the air conditioner in the bedroom is broken. It makes a terrible sound and blows hot air.

Time has stopped and it makes me panic. I cannot sleep. I walk into Luke's room and remember another time I felt that everything had stopped. We were waiting for Luke to be born. He was two weeks overdue. I couldn't sleep at night; I was too uncomfortable. I tossed and turned and periodically lumbered to the bathroom. I knew I was disturbing Keith, he often joked or complained about my fitfulness, but I was too miserable to care. One night Keith turned to me and said, "Would it help if I read to you?" I was touched: Keith hardly ever read. I handed him the collection of stories by Colette by my side of the bed and he took the book, sat up in bed, and read, slowly and carefully, occasionally putting his hand on my belly or stroking my hair. I don't remember the story; I remember watching him read. He finished the story at dawn. I said I still didn't feel sleepy but felt so incredibly tired. Maybe a beer would help. So we shared a beer and watched the sun come up. We held hands. It didn't matter that it was morning; we were waiting for something that transcended the limits of night and day. We watched the dawn and then fell asleep.

I am haunted by the thought that we are waiting now, waiting for something equally monumental. And now there is no pregnant belly to watch move.

Last night Keith said to me, "It is a very strong instinct, the feeling that you want to reach a resolution. Dying is a temptation. You and Luke keep reminding me that dying is not the solution . . . but it never goes away."

I worry about Keith's depression. I am bitchy angry—aggressive, hostile. But Keith seems to be beyond that. He is so angry he is silent and withdrawn. When his father was noncommittal and almost uninterested in helping us out financially (his uncle never responded), it was as if Keith had been stabbed, and now he has retired to lick his wounds. But it seems to me that his wounds are not healing naturally. He is trying to heal them with determination. And it is just too exhausting.

August 15

We had a heavenly two-week vacation in Germantown. We became whole and well as a family. We saw nobody, we had no schedule. The two weeks passed like one long summer's day that was ours to enjoy. Layers of tension fell away. We were self-indulgent and felt no guilt. So hungry for peace and space.

With no one else around to serve as a contrast with Keith, he seemed healthy in his way. He gained weight and regained his sense of humor. Any anxieties he had about running away and being isolated from the world disappeared after the first week, when Dick called to say that they needed music for Calvin Klein's new commercials. We giggled every evening when Keith beeped in to get our messages and there would be Dick's voice describing his ideas for this manic, insane commercial.

The first few days in Germantown it seemed it would rain forever. A baptism of rain. We played quietly inside with Luke. Looked out the window and watched the swampy patch at the bottom of the lawn become a rushing stream. Put on boots in the afternoon and waded through the mud to the chickenhouse to feed the chickens, Luke splashing in the puddles and shaking water off branches. I put Luke to sleep listening to the sound of the rain on the roof. I curled up in bed and felt as if we were all on a ship, destination unknown.

Then it cleared and grew hot. Keith shaved outside in the sun, Luke bringing him bowls of water. We lounged on blankets. We packed picnic lunches and drove to the river to swim, Keith's music playing on the car cassette player. Keith swam. Keith and I held Luke as he waded in over his head.

In the late afternoon Keith and I sat outside. We watched Luke chase the chickens—around the house into the woods, giggling, screeching really, at the silly birds. Trying to corner them. Trying to get them to fly. Luke's chicken dance. Keith and I laughed. Luke continued until the sun went down. Then we herded the chickens into the chickenhouse and went in to eat dinner.

After dinner I started the dishes and Keith and Luke did their dance through the house. The pipes knocked rhythmically shaking the house. Keith told Luke it was the Uugha-Uugha Man. There was a picture of an Indian with fruit balanced on his head on the wall of the stairwell. Keith and Luke bowed down in front of it and then gyrated through the house—"uugha, uugha"—waving their hands in the air. I stopped the dishes and took Luke upstairs to brush his teeth. The pipes knocked again. Luke collapsed in laughter as Keith started dancing in the hall, "Uugha, uugha." Luke went to bed giggling.

And one night Keith reached for me. It didn't matter that he never entered me, that the conventional sex act ended when he reached for the condoms. We needed and wanted each other. Something was acknowledged. We had connected. We held each other through the night.

When we returned to New York and I walked into our apartment I was horrified. Every cell in my body rebelled at the thought of spending another winter in this apartment. I felt our apartment was dangerous, haunted. We must get out now, quickly, before it was too late. We'd come so far in the last ten months. We needed a new apartment because our life had entered a new phase. The memories of last winter were too vivid here. If we didn't move we would be sucked back to where we were last winter. We made plans to move into a friend's sublet on Twenty-first Street.

If only Keith and I could open up in this apartment as we did in the country. I find it impossible. I'm starting to feel on the defensive again—battening down my emotional hatches, closing the storm windows.

I lie in bed with my head on Keith's shoulder. Sometimes we go to sleep holding hands. But we aren't touching more than that. Germantown is remembered like a dream.

Keith is working on the commercial. That seems to be all that is on his mind. I am worrying about him and the move. Enveloped in my bubble of anxiety all day. Seems I can only relax when Luke and Keith are home, asleep.

Keith's doing the commercial has taken the edge off our financial situation. We will have money to move. We'll have money to get through December. We don't think about buying a new apartment now. These days a sublet for two years seems like forever. And what we do not say to each other is that we may need the money from this apartment's sale to live on. I will not say that out loud because I must not think it. Keith is well enough to work. He will always be well enough to work. But somehow Keith's working doesn't seem important anymore. Home is what matters now. We must move on and make our new home better. But our doubts are numbing us. I can't take in the fact that we are leaving our home of ten years. Neither of us is enthusiastic; neither of us is nostalgic. I am numb. I will not allow myself any sentimental feelings. Moving is a necessity now. I am impatient and afraid during the day. I am only reflective when Luke and Keith are asleep.

In the middle of the night I walk barefoot around the perimeter of our apartment. I look at Keith asleep in our bed in one room and at Luke asleep in his crib in the other. I feel proud and content. I get in bed with my arms folded under my head and stare at the ceiling. I imagine I am floating above the apartment like a protective figurehead on the bow of a ship. I feel peaceful knowing that there is one unshakable given among all of life's uncertainties: I will do anything to protect my family.

We went out to dinner for our wedding anniversary. Extremely peaceful and subdued. No philosophical observations, few mentions of Keith's being sick. We simply said that we were glad we had each other. I told Keith that I loved him and admired him more than ever. I spoke sincerely.

It is a gratifying feeling—knowing that we have come together as a family again. With the strength and comfort we get from each other we can face reality better. I no longer pray for Keith to get well—I pray that he doesn't get worse.

August 28

Today I am remembering the game my mind played last September when we didn't know what was wrong with Keith. I would be walking down the street. The air was cool and clear and I could smell and feel things as if they were from a different place, a different dimension. There was dry electricity in the air. As people approached and walked past me I would look at them and decide if they were dying or not, and I could really tell—I knew. By the time they had passed me on the street their fates were sealed. I guessed at how long they were going to live. I never questioned my conclusions. And I never questioned why I was playing this morbid game. I could see how much life reserve every person had—if he or she was using up a diminishing supply, fighting to stay alive, or flourishing and healthy. I had x-ray vision. I knew strangers' health. Maybe I was going crazy, entering an underside of life.

Now that I know Keith is sick, I am aware of a new dimension, the one of "vibrations"—helpful, hurtful, soothing, destructive. They surround people and color situations. They permeate space and time; they enable me to relax or make me tense and angry. My family is being hurt or it is safe and comfortable. Our life is progressing or it is being thwarted and damaged. There's something primitive, almost animal-like in the way I experience everything in terms of how it affects my family. Like a wild dog protecting her den.

September 5

Keith's working makes me anxious. I am anxious about him in the professional world, where he has to pretend he is well. I worry about his handling the stress inherent in the charade.

But perhaps I'm not giving Keith enough credit. He seems to be enjoying working—and buzzing around town in Champagne Car. And he is working with Dick, who knows he is sick. I think it gives Keith some security being with someone who shares his secret. He came home the other night and said, "Dick keeps trying to get me to sit down, he keeps asking me if I want to sit down. He is always following me around with this chair." He said it with annoyance, but I could tell he was touched.

September 15

My brother, Robert, married his girlfriend, Annie, in her family's home in Syracuse. We drove to the wedding. We left on

Keith's birthday, which was all right, a relief in a way—I had been very uncertain about how to celebrate it. Luke and I gave him our gifts in the morning, then we left on the drive. It was our first long trip since Keith had gotten sick, and it took a lot of mental preparation. Keith was worried about feeling like an outcast. Or maybe he was worried about proving that he is one of the living. It's hard for Keith to make new forays into the outside world when they entail seeing people who haven't seen him in a long time. I get anxious too. I feel they're going to be comparing the Keith they knew before he got sick with Keith now. My personal frame of reference has shrunk: I compare Keith now with Keith in the terrible winter months, and all seems well to me. I don't want anything to shatter my equilibrium. It's taken us a long time to be healthy as a family again.

The wedding was wonderful, almost exhilarating, in all the warm, good ways weddings should be. Keith had written Robert and Annie a song, which he, I and my sisters performed as a toast at the prenuptial dinner. It was an upbeat, pop-tune-type song called "Lifted by the Power of Love." My sisters and I sang harmony on the chorus, sort of like the Supremes.

Luke is refusing to allow us to leave him at nursery school. I think they are starting to label him a difficult child and I'm beginning to feel that I don't want to leave him there. He comes home and sees boxes being packed. I tell myself that is why he's so clingy. But fall is in the air and I keep thinking that Luke feels it too and remembers. The air gets cooler, you put sweaters on, and first your Daddy and then your Mommy disappears. And when they come back they come back different.

FALL

Keith has started seeing spots before his eyes—floaters. He went to an eye doctor, Dr. Christel, recommended by Dr. Davis. She said it was genetic, something about the jelly on his retina shrinking. She said that the floaters would go away. They haven't.

He came home from his therapist and said he didn't feel safe driving. Floaters come and go across his field of vision, creating blind spots.

I've started painting the new apartment. Decided to make friends with this feeling of panic. It is getting familiar.

When friends come to help me paint I get nervous and start feeling that I want to be alone. So I've been working alone and sometimes I get a little crazy. I wonder where Keith is. I say to myself he is home babysitting Luke but my stomach starts cramping with panic.

Then I start feeling sorry for myself. Keith and I always used to paint together and we will never paint a home together again. I start to think of the future. If Keith has a future he will need my constant support and this is too hard. I remember Keith's support of my flute playing. His caring. Recording my concerts for me. His praise. The dinners he cooked for me when I was pregnant. I look out the window and start to cry. The way he could always talk me out of my tears. My stomach tightens. It is O.K., I tell myself, it is going to be all right. I decide to wash the windows and scrub every inch of the floors before moving day, even if it means staying up all night.

October 3

Someone in my support group said that his lover had had floaters and had gone to four doctors before they found an infection. By the time they caught it he had lost most of the sight in his left eye. We made an appointment with the doctor who had found this man's infection.

The appointment was on the morning of my birthday. The doctor was very thorough. He said the same thing as Dr. Christel—that he couldn't find any infection. We didn't feel very relieved. Keith says he feels as if he is going crazy, that the doctors don't know what they are saying. Keith says that the spots are worse and he is seeing bright flashes of light.

After the trip to the eye doctor I went over to the new apartment to do some more painting. When I came home Keith and Luke had made me a wonderful birthday party. Just the three of us. Festive and cozy.

If we wake up before Luke, Keith and I read the newspaper

in bed. This morning Keith read the paper before me. He was busy with Luke when I saw the picture of our friend Charles Ward in the obituaries. AIDS. I didn't know what to say to Keith because I knew that he had seen it and he hadn't said anything to me. I just said, "This is terrible." Keith said that he had seen the picture and until he started reading he thought it was a review of his latest performance.

I felt sick. I remembered Charles in our home and his phone calls. He was so reckless, almost self-destructive, but very gifted and intelligent. And now all that talent and energy are gone. We hadn't seen him since he moved to California four years ago. Keith said tonight that he feels like calling someone who was close to him to find out what his last years were like. I can't answer him in anything but platitudes.

That night Keith and I talked. I said I was terrified of his going into the hospital for treatment for his eyes. Keith said he was terrified of going blind. Keith asked me if I thought we should cancel the movers. If he was going blind, how could he live in an apartment where he didn't know where the bathroom was? He also said that he had a growth on his thigh that hurt.

I said that we shouldn't cancel anything until we knew what was wrong. I decided to steel myself for the move. I felt that my family was a triangle and I was the top point, supporting the other two points. The image made me feel unbearably lonely.

October 7

We've moved. I was so nervous I sat and smoked while Luke ate his breakfast at the Empire. Keith was supervising the movers. That night in our new home we felt excited and proud. We were self-contained in a new place. It as a light, heady feeling, like being in the country. We had done it.

October 19

Been in this apartment about two weeks now. I've started getting depressed and angry. Feeling exhausted. The wedding, Keith's eyes, Luke not adjusting to nursery school, turning thirty-three, and moving have all left me exhausted and wondering, "Where am I?"

The furniture is in place; only a few boxes are left unpacked. Physically we have settled in. From the living-room window we can see the sun set over the Hudson. Sitting up in our bed we can see it rise in the east. And it is quiet here. We get in bed at night and say that it is like the country—no trucks, no fights on the street.

But Keith and I cannot sleep. I fall asleep and wake a couple of hours later and roam the apartment. I find Keith in the rocking chair in the living room. I lie near him on the couch. I look at the river. I look at him. All we say to each other is "You can't sleep either?"

We feel the fall. Winter is coming. We are silent. We are remembering. We are apprehensive. In the dark we feel what we repress during the day—our fear. It's a fear that comes from knowing that, when all is said and done, our fate is out of our hands. We are scared—terrified really—of winter's coming. Winter represents the unknown. We don't talk to each other.

Sometimes I wish Keith would go to bed and I could be alone—I can't stand seeing him rocking in the dark. At around 4 A.M. we give up. We turn on the television and watch *Ben Casey* reruns. When the sky starts to lighten we feel ashamed of the glow from the television. We go to bed around 5 or 6 A.M.

The air is getting thinner; it is getting cold at night. We aren't talking to each other and I cannot stand our not talking.

* * *

Keith's growth is only a boil, treatable with antibiotics.

October 26

Keith and I have started seeing Susan together. We know we have to talk. And it has helped take the lid off the pressure cooker. We can let our defenses down there. But I have my doubts about it—it makes me nervous. I guess I just don't like hearing Keith talk about being sick, worried, afraid. Dying.

He says it in her office. He says that he feels he has let me down. He says that he hates himself. I cannot listen. He says that he wants to take care of his family. That that is what is important to him. I feel myself tense and sweating. Please don't say that, that isn't what is important, I can take care of us, just say that you will live. Don't say that you don't want to be dependent, don't say that you feel like a burden, please don't say that you are scared of dying. Say that you will live.

The antibiotic for Keith's boil is making him sick. He's lost his appetite and his energy. Dr. Davis is trying to get some AZT for him.

Yesterday, Dr. Amchi, the Tibetan doctor, was in New York. Keith's cousin John picked up Keith and me in a taxi and took us to a tenement on the Lower East Side. Keith wasn't supposed to have any caffeine or exert himself before having his pulse read, but we had to climb six flights of stairs to the apartment. The Tibetan who owned the apartment ushered us in. Dr. Amchi was sitting cross-legged on a small bed, wearing a polo shirt and felt skirt. A short stocky man with a tremendously broad forehead and high cheekbones, pointed ears, and extremely intelligent eyes. I felt we were very much in another world—a comfortable, peaceful one where we were the aliens. Dr. Amchi read Keith's pulse, looked at his knees, and then touched a place on Keith's chest. He gave an amazingly accurate picture of the history of Keith's illness. In Tibetan (there was a translator) he said that Keith had had the illness for five or six years and that it had first manifested itself in his large intestine, with diarrhea. He was right on. He told Keith that he should relax, stay warm, get some exercise, and have confidence, that he had seen men in worse shape than Keith and they had gotten better. Then we had tea. He said that the medicine he was prescribing would be ready to be picked up in the morning.

When we got home from the Tibetan doctor Luke and Keith napped and I started to read the AZT release form that Keith had gotten from Dr. Davis. Keith wanted me to read it because he had been frightened by the description of its side effects. Terrifying. I feel we are entering a twilight zone of not knowing which is worse, the illness or the cure. Such an awful frustration, not knowing what to do. Western medicine, Eastern medicine—what will happen if Keith takes them together? What will happen if he doesn't? What will happen?

After Luke was in bed that night we talked. Keith told me he has decided to go ahead and give the Tibetan drugs a try. Once Dr. Davis gets the AZT for him, he can think about whether to continue with Dr. Amchi's medicines or not. He'll see how he feels.

I wish I could have complete faith in the Tibetan treatment. Dr. Amchi has such a wise, intelligent, compassionate aura, and the treatment sounds so simple and straightforward. If it works the way he says it will, we won't have to worry about whether to take the AZT. But something has to start working. Keith has been looking very white, and he's barely eating these days.

We drove down to pick up the medicine this morning at nine, Luke sleepy and wrapped in a blanket, I jumpy from all the coffee I had drunk in preparation for the six flights of stairs. Right at nine, as we had planned, someone threw the keys to the front door out the window. I ran up the stairs. Dr. Amchi was sitting on the bed with his prayer beads. Another Tibetan man was just out of the shower, wrapped in a towel. The room was sunny and peaceful. It smelled of tea and toast.

Then we went to the South Street Seaport. It was deserted; it hadn't opened yet. We had a picnic breakfast on the pier.

October 27

Keith has started taking the Tibetan drugs. He's determined to give them a good shot. Immediately he began to look better to me. His color improved. But they are making him sick to his stomach.

When I look at the ribavirin in the fridge I long for an established course of action, an easy answer. But the choices are Keith's. Only he can judge how his body responds. I wish I could help him with the choices. After all, like me, I'm sure he doesn't want to get too lonely.

It's the first chilly, rainy day we've had in a long time. Keith took Luke to play at my parents' house in Brooklyn. I'm feeling that it's nice in this home. Made phone calls, did laundry, and played my flute.

November 2

Rachel's baby, Aaron, was born Tuesday evening. Wednesday morning Keith suggested that we take off for Washington to see him. I was wonderfully surprised by Keith's suggesting this spontaneous adventure. I felt exhilarated packing our overnight bags.

But as we started to drive through New Jersey Keith suggested that we park in Newark and fly. That sounded crazy to me. Then he said that he had a huge floater in his right eye and everything was distorting around it. He didn't feel safe driving. I drove.

Keith called Dr. Christel from Washington and made an appointment for Monday. When we got home Thursday, Keith called Dr. Davis to say that he was losing the sight in his right eye. Dr. Davis said he would dilate the eye and take a look the next day, Halloween, a year to the day since Keith had left for Europe.

Friday morning before Keith's appointment with Dr. Davis was horrible. I felt torn between Luke and Keith—trying to be calm and cheerful for Luke, trying to be supportive to Keith, losing all sense of what I was feeling, suppressing my panic. Luke and I bought Halloween masks and made jack o'lanterns.

Dr. Davis didn't find any infection. He saw a large floater and said it would go away. Keith came home feeling as if he were going crazy. Was everyone lying to him? Why couldn't he see out of his right eye? Dr. Davis told Keith that he was dressing up that night as a stewardess for the Halloween parade. Keith, feeling angry, said that Dr. Davis seemed more concerned about finding the surgical tape to hold his false eyelashes on than about figuring out what was wrong with Keith's eyes.

That night we went to Brooklyn to have dinner with my father. Mother was in Washington helping Rachel with her new baby. Luke and I took our masks (Luke is a cat, I'm a butterfly) and a jack o'lantern. Keith took the electric blanket. As soon as we arrived Keith plugged the blanket in, lay down on the window seat, and went to sleep until dinner. I think it was a slight shock to my father, but soon it began to seem quite cozy and normal. My father served huge gin martinis. Daddy was, in Keith's words, like Ebenezer Scrooge the morning after. It was a Halloween party.

So depressed this weekend. It's the anniversary of Keith's leaving for Europe. I tell myself we've come a long way in a year. I tell myself that since Keith has outlived the English doctors' prognosis perhaps he will outlive everyone's prognosis. But I don't feel optimistic. I feel we are entering a twilight zone of symptoms that are not cut and dried. Nobody knows what to do or what will happen. We are all floundering.

Keith can never get warm. He is always bundled in long underwear, sweaters, parkas. And it isn't even winter yet.

I yelled and screamed and sobbed this morning. Major emotional cleaning. Jealous of my sister—jealous that she had my family's attention when my life was so scary and undefined. Angry that I couldn't stay in bed alone, *alone* . . . angry that I had lost my center because Rachel had had a baby, because Keith couldn't see, because Luke was cutting up as a result of all the excitement and tension. I had lost my footing and I was damned if I was going to try to get it back before I had been a baby myself for a few hours.

We went to the top of the Empire State Building. It was a damp, cloudy, blowy day and I kept wanting to cry. After we came home I got it together to go to Macy's while Luke was asleep. Found some clothes I liked. In the dressing room I took off my clothes and stood between the opposing walls of mirrors. I was startled by the length of my hair. It had never been so long. It fell way past my shoulders to my waist, curtaining the curve of the small of my back. Under those horrible fluorescent lights I thought that I looked beautiful. It was such a surprise to think that. Not having a sex life is doing some strange things.

November 3

Keith came home from Dr. Christel's this afternoon teary and scared. She found a sign of infection. She thinks the floaters may have been a warning sign of the infection. She said she doesn't feel qualified to make a diagnosis without a second opinion. Keith is going to see another doctor, Dr. Levin, at eight tomorrow morning. Pure panic and dread have settled like stones in my stomach—and a feeling that is like homesickness, terrible homesickness. I want my Keith close. I feel that something awful is going to take him away from his home, my home, our home. I cry whenever no one is around. Riding alone in the elevator I hold the door half open so it won't go, so I'll have a little more time alone to cry.

November 4

At seven-forty-five, I drove Keith up to Dr. Levin's office at Eighty-eighth and Park. Robert had arrived at seven-thirty to babysit. It was a dark, wet, quiet drive. I dropped Keith off and went home. Two hours when time didn't pass because the hard tightness in my stomach never got worse or better. Luke kept asking for his Daddy. Keith came home at eleven. Dr. Levin said that he has an infection that is in his blood, but he doesn't know what it is yet. He needs to have blood drawn. All the damage is permanent. Tomorrow the doctor wants to do a test at Mt. Sinai to see how extensive the damage is.

Luke walked in on Keith and me in tears. He came over and gave us each a kiss. Then he acted like a banshee the rest of the morning.

The three of us went out and did errands. Even though he can't drive, Keith likes to feel in control. It was important to him to do the banking. I was weepy and tense.

Keith and I took a nap together. I felt much better after we held each other. Keith felt so good. Keith told me to take care of myself, that Luke needed me. He said to try not to get too involved, that I shouldn't panic, that Luke needs a calm person to take his cues from. I told him that was impossible.

After nap time we all went down to Dr. Davis's so they could take Keith's blood. Luke charmed the office.

November 6

The tests at Mt. Sinai were to see the extent of the damage from the infection—how much of Keith's retina was still working, responding to light. They dilated Keith's eyes and then put electrodes on his eyeballs. A computer recorded his retina's response.

Dr. Levin seemed very concerned and caring. He said that AIDS has opened up a whole new field in ophthalmology. A year ago people were going blind and doctors didn't know what to do. Testing Keith would help them know a little more.

The doctor who administered the test was much more blunt. He said that Keith was the second person he had seen with this kind of infection. Of course the first man went totally blind.

After the test Keith said he wanted to take me out to dinner. He said he wanted it to be a real date, without my worrying about driving. He hired a car. Annie came to sit. It was cold and rainy. We were shy with each other, quiet really. So many things we couldn't begin to say out loud. Tentative and nervous.

It is the middle of the night. I want to cry. I want to talk to Keith and he is sleeping. It was the car he hired. That gesture has broken my heart. Does he know how hard it is for me to drive him? I hate driving Keith, knowing that he cannot drive a car.

He said to me tonight, "If I had known in August it was the

last time I would drive down a country road I would have appreciated it more. I wish I had known."

Keith loves to drive. I've often wondered what it must be like for Keith never to have known how to run, how to race downhill, how to be effortlessly mobile. It must be awful, because the pleasure Keith felt driving a car has always been so intense, so appreciative of motion, that it speaks of the lack.

I remember Keith driving us around Denver in the middle of the night. The motion of driving always inspired Keith. He loved the control it gave him. Keith explored in cars. Driving was both a catharsis and an open door for him. Whenever we felt trapped in the city Keith would say, "I just want to drive on a country road."

Twice we drove across country to New York from Denver. The first time was to get to our wedding at my grandmother's home in Vermont—my wedding dress and his wedding suit hanging in the back of a "drive-away" telephone repair truck. The second time was in our orange van, driving our furniture and large possessions to New York, after I had relented and agreed to join Keith in New York. That trip we drove seventy-two hours without stopping. The late mornings and early afternoons were hard, but the nights were heaven. Three A.M. in the middle of Kansas. The radio on and windows open. Alone on the road. I sat with my feet on the dashboard, my hand out the window. Keith would reach over and touch my hair; I'd reach over and massage his shoulders. Completely self-contained.

We used to go to my family's place in Maine in the spring or fall. We would leave the city at midnight and Keith would drive until dawn. We took a tape player with us. At around two or three I'd go to sleep on the back seat and listen to Keith playing tapes of his music or singing new melodies to himself.

Keith has CMV-induced retinitis. He needs to be treated with DHPG, administered intravenously in the hospital—a three-week treatment.

We spent Friday waiting for a hospital bed—really scared. The weather is cold and raining. English weather. London all over again. If Keith goes in the hospital will he ever get out? Does someone know something we don't? (Someone must, I thought. Keith is going blind.) I couldn't bear to think of us losing control of this disease.

We waited and we got ready. And Keith amazed me. He worked out how to hold his own.

He made sure there was a note from Dr. Christel saying that Luke could visit him at any hour. He packed his radio/cassette player and tapes. He called Wayne and told him that I would need him and to make sure I used him.

When Keith arrived in his room it looked as if the former occupant had not left according to plan—his razor and shampoo were still in the medicine cabinet. I washed out the cabinet and sink. I brought the portable heater, the down quilt, some of Luke's drawings (one strategically placed over the picture of the Virgin Mary), magazines, food (he had a refrigerator in his room), and framed photographs. We made a nest for Keith. And the doctors started the DHPG IV.

The first two evenings at home I felt that I was being subjected to a new torture called Having Your Child Mirror All the Feelings You Are Trying to Hide. Luke kept saying, "I want Daddy to come home. I miss Daddy. When is Daddy coming home?" And I would say, "Daddy is coming home soon. . . . He needs the medicine in the hospital to get better." I kept wondering how convincing I was. I know it couldn't have helped Luke much that I gave in to him so often those first few days. If he didn't want a shampoo I wouldn't insist. If he didn't want to go to bed I'd let him stay up with me watching TV. I suppose he was more of a comfort to me than I was to him. I couldn't sleep. I felt alone. I couldn't relax. Is the door locked? Is that Luke waking up?

Early Sunday morning Luke and I took the bus to St. Margaret's. Luke lay on the hospital bed next to Keith. He played with the buttons that made Keith's bed go up and down and with the remote television controls. He thought hospital beds were great.

That first visit Luke cried when it was time to leave. He couldn't accept the fact that Keith couldn't come with us. Now he knows the ritual of Keith's walking us to the elevator, IV pole in hand, and the kisses good-bye before the elevator comes.

Keith can't accept the inevitable next step, having a catheter put in his chest. How can he have a brace on his leg and a tube coming out of his chest? he asks. So unfair.

I don't know what to say to him. I can't listen to his objections, his fears—I'm having enough trouble accepting it myself. I'm short with him. We fight on the phone.

I had heard about Hickmans in my support group. I remember being horrified at the idea of needing so many drugs that you had to have a special apparatus to get them into your body. The thought was repugnant to me. But I saw in my group that people got used to them. One woman said she and her husband had gone on a camping trip. Every afternoon she hung his IV bag of drugs from the ceiling of their car while her husband lay across the back seat. I knew we could get used to it too.

Keith is reacting to it as a physical disfigurement. What upsets me is that I see it as another stage in the progression of the disease; it represents another stage in what seems, these days, to be a losing battle. First the Hickman, then the wheelchair.

I don't want to be pulled under, I don't want to feel defeated, just when I had begun to feel good about how we are managing.

I find it hard to play a supportive role with Keith when I am suffering from my own fears and disappointments.

Keith says he won't let them take him to surgery until he knows what kind of catheter they are going to put in. Keith wants an Infusaport, which lies under the skin. Dr. Davis wants him to have a Hickman, which has a rubber tube sticking out. Keith argues that he takes baths with Luke and a tube coming out of his chest would confuse and upset his son.

Keith said he spent Dr. Davis's morning visit crying in Dr. Davis's arms.

November 14

He went to surgery.

I went down to the hospital at five, which is when I had been told Keith would be back in his room. He wasn't. The floor nurse called down to the recovery room to find out where he was. She told me they were deciding whether or not to take Keith to Intensive Care. I panicked, called Annie, and she said she would be right down. I waited in Keith's hospital room. The surgeon called on the phone and he said he would be right up to tell me what happened. I sat in Keith's room shaking, old terror coming back.

The surgeon arrived and started drawing diagrams of a heart. I couldn't figure out what he was doing. He said that Keith's heartbeat became irregular when they pushed the end of the catheter in. Said he'd take me to see Keith. Annie arrived as we were leaving for the recovery room.

Keith was awake and coherent. Plugged into a heart monitor. Made sense to me that anyone's heart would start to spasm. The cardiologist came and went. Nothing to worry about, might correct itself. Keith was moved to the Cardiac Care Unit for the night. Annie and I went out to dinner. Keith was too drugged to talk when we checked in on him before going home. But he looked O.K. to me. Drugged and sleeping. So reminiscent of England—hospitals at night and lots of drugs.

Keith's heart reverted back to normal while they finished putting the catheter in this morning. They put in an Infusaport. The surgeon is proud of it. He said, "We really pulled one over on Dr. Davis."

I have a terrible cold. I took a day off from visiting the hospital. Wayne took Luke to see his Daddy. Such a grownup boy walking out the door with Wayne.

November 16

The Tibetan doctor, Dr. Amchi, came to visit Keith in his hospital room: a short man in a down jacket, knit watchcap, and cheap oxfords walking through the door of Keith's room with his secretary, the translator, and John. Dr. Traube (the assisting surgeon) and another young St. Margaret's doctor were there out of curiosity. Dr. Amchi took off his jacket (I hung it in Keith's closet . . . how do you play hostess in a hospital room?) and sat down at Keith's bedside in maroon and yellow robes. Wonderful. He felt Keith's pulse at both wrists. He asked for the light to be shone on Keith's eyes so he could examine them. He touched Keith's feet. Then he said that he thought Keith was better than when he had seen him before. He said that if Keith continued the medicine he prescribed, followed the diet he had given him a month ago, and avoids sex for seven months, Keith would feel noticeably better and could even be cured in a year. He said that Keith should continue taking the

Western medicine, but take the Tibetan medicine too, at least an hour before or after it.

I walked the entourage to the elevator. Dr. Amechi said that nothing could be done about Keith's eyes.

November 19

Keith is going to come home soon. He will need a visiting nurse for a couple of hours every day to help him administer the DHPG.

Luke and I have adjusted to Keith's being away. I've put the curtains up, put pictures on the bedroom walls, hired a maid for one morning a week.

The thought of Keith's coming home scares me.

November 26

Keith came home Saturday. Pat, Larry, and Brandon came over to be with Luke while I went with Wayne to pick Keith up. It was a beautiful day. Everything seemed shimmery and sparkly. Keith was so appreciative of his home, of being home. And Luke seemed so pleased, not frantic, about Keith's arrival. Luke and I had baked a cake together to celebrate Daddy's coming home. We served it to Keith in his bed. Everything seemed good.

But at dinner that night I got drunk because whenever Keith looked at me it seemed as though his eyes weren't seeing me, as though they weren't connecting with me, as though they were part of a mask. Keith is a lot weaker and whiter than before he went into the hospital, and his eyes aren't any better. And nobody is saying whether they will get better, or stay the same, or get worse.

* * *

There have been some difficult times these first couple of days with Keith home. I've felt trapped . . . felt that everyone needed caring for . . . needed me. I've had moments of real panic and claustrophobia. The second night Keith was home he was throwing up in the bathroom while I was putting Luke to bed. Luke kept asking, "What's Daddy doing?"

But I like smelling Keith near me in bed in the middle of the night. And having the visiting nurse seems O.K. Somehow it makes me feel that some of the pressure is off me.

Monday our friend David took Keith down to his appointment with Dr. Davis. He came home with his first three bottles of AZT. Dr. Davis had gotten it in earlier, but decided to wait awhile before giving it to Keith because he's not sure how it will interact with the DHPG. With the DHPG the risks of AZT are even greater than what the release form says, so it's hard to feel optimistic about his taking it. We're both nervous.

That evening I was leafing through one of the magazines Keith had brought home from the hospital with him. There was a double-page fund-raising picture for the American Foundation for AIDS Research, showing a group of celebrities wearing buttons that say "We Care." Dick was one of the group. I showed it to Keith. He burst into tears. When I asked him why he was crying, he said, "It's so naïve." More and more we feel that we inhabit a world that healthy people, even with the best of intentions, know nothing about.

November 29

Thanksgiving we went to Pat and Larry's for dinner. I was in heaven—feeling cared for, cooked for. This year I had sense enough not to try to do anything at home; I knew it would have been too much. And Keith seemed to enjoy being out in the world, seeing his sister and her family.

After we got home at eight-thirty the nurse arrived as planned. Everything was working out. Luke and I went out and bought cookies while Keith got hooked up to his IV.

The day after Thanksgiving was a beautiful sunny day. Luke and I went to the park in the morning. In the afternoon Keith went out, by himself, to Dr. Davis's to have the catheter stitches taken out. Luke went down for his nap. The house was clean. Life seemed good. I made some tea and waited for Keith to get home.

Keith walked in the door and said that Dr. Davis thought he was a marvel, doing amazingly well. I looked at him and said, "Your shirt is wet. Did he take out the stitches? What is making your shirt wet?" I picked up Keith's tee shirt and his chest wound was open and there was his Infusaport and the darkness of deep in his chest and this is not right. "Call Dr. Davis. Go right back to Dr. Davis. Should I wake Luke and drive you? Be careful. You really think you can manage?"

Everything after that I hate, hate, hate, because it was so needless and harmful and should never have happened.

Keith made it to Dr. Davis's office. When I called his office they said that Keith was on his way to St. Margaret's emergency room. Then Keith called to say that he couldn't get a cab. I woke Luke and we drove down to pick Keith up. I told Luke we had to rush because this was an emergency. Luke kept saying, "It's O.K.," over and over. Dropped Keith off at the emergency-room entrance, parked the car, and rushed in, pushing Luke in his stroller. "Can't bring a child in here." Dr. Traube arrived and said it was O.K. to bring Luke in. . . . Curtains drawn around Keith, I realizing this is no place for a child. Going home without Keith.

Mother came over to watch Luke and I went back to the hospital. Keith was in a room down the hall from the one he had left less than a week ago. We joked about the malpractice suit we could bring against . . . whom? The surgeon? Dr. Davis? Did Dr. Davis take the stitches out too soon? Or should the surgeon never have put the Infusaport in in the first place? We found out later that the reason Dr. Davis had wanted the Hickman was that AIDS patients' wounds heal poorly. The surgeon obviously didn't know that. The end result of all of this was that Keith was going to have a Hickman catheter, the one he had fought so hard against, put in the next morning. There was Virgin Mary staring down on Keith in his bed, only this time I didn't have anything to cover her up with. (Keith said it was just as well; maybe that's why everything had gone wrong before.) I had brought only Keith's bare essentials, toothbrush and quilt from home. His room looked cold. And I was overcome by anger. Why was this happening? What kind of outrage is this? Why did Keith, an immune-deficient person, have to hail a cab and ride around Manhattan with a gaping hole in his chest?

In the end it is out of my hands. He's in a hospital bed with other people taking care of him, and I'm left angry and worried. Huge temptation to say fuck it all. Keith was joking about it— he wanted to make sure I knew who to sue if he died in surgery the next day . . . think how rich I'd be.

I hate hospitals, I hate the medical profession. Keith lying in bed facing a nonworking TV and a picture of an old woman with a halo around her head. Hooked up to an IV, with no food except the deli sandwich and orange juice I had brought him.

I took Luke to the park the next morning. No more dramas and tears over surgery like the last time. I made Keith promise he would ask Dr. Traube to call me after it was over. Dr. Traube called around one. Everything was fine. Luke wanted to talk to him and did. I don't think Luke had any idea who he was talking to.

I left Luke at Pat and Larry's after his nap and went to see Keith. His room was dark. He still had his surgical hat on. His dinner tray was on the bed table next to him, smelling foul. No one had pulled the sheets up. He looked as though he had been parked, not put to bed. He was in pain. He was clutching the phone, which was on his stomach. I guess he had put it there when he had called me two hours earlier to say he was back in his room. He said it hurt.

I asked the nurse to page Dr. Traube to ask if Keith could be given more pain medication. They brought him Valium. He had some water. I arranged his water and orange juice on the bed table so he could reach them. I left as they were about to give him more drugs.

November 30

Feeling bereft. Everyone's away for Thanksgiving weekend and I can't find a babysitter. Luke and I did laundry and then went to the playground. Keith called. Sounded as if he were doing all right. During nap time I vacuumed and washed my hair and practiced.

After Luke woke up I began to feel better. We drew and painted and danced and laughed. I felt strong and secure in my home. Then, after supper, Keith called to say he was miserable and had a fever of 103.5.

I want him here, home. I feel that it is dangerous out there, in that hospital. Come home. We have the eye drugs, we have AZT. Why can't he come home? Do it here?

Keith called at 7 A.M. Said he had been delirious all night with a fever of 104. I was too sleepy to panic. I called Robert to ask him to watch Luke while I went to the hospital. Keith's fever was down to 101. I gave him a sponge bath. Left him clean, powdered, and comfortable. Luke was upset and confused by Robert's babysitting and not being able to take the bus to the hospital to see Daddy as I had said we would. Instead when I got home we did errands and went out to lunch. After his nap I took him up to Pat and Larry's for the evening.

I arrived at St. Margaret's around seven that night. Keith said that he had called the nurse at six to come take his temperature because he was burning up. She had said it wasn't time to take temperatures, so he took it himself. It was 104.5. As I sponged his back and forehead he felt so hot it seemed as though steam should be rising from his skin.

Dr. Davis arrived soon after I did. His demeanor was reassuring and confident. The fever would go away. It was the flu, or a reaction to the anesthesia, or a reaction to the interaction of the anesthesia and AZT. Keith had brought his bottle of AZT to the hospital with him. Dr. Davis told me to take it home.

Keith told Dr. Davis his gripes, beginning with the nun who arrived in the morning and asked him what kind of prayer he would like her to say for him. Keith asked for a hopeful prayer. She said it was hard to find a hopeful prayer for patients with AIDS. Then there was Dr. Traube telling him just before surgery how lucky he was to have Dr. Venk operating on him because most surgeons won't touch someone with AIDS. And the nurses on the floor (an orthopedic floor) being insensitive to the importance of a fever in an AIDS patient, not knowing it can shoot up almost instantly.

It is cruel that Keith has to defend and explain himself when he is sick and suffering.

Dr. Davis said that Dr. Venk was being reprimanded "in a financial way" for putting in the Infusaport. Keith and I must take some action on this mix-up. Not only is it wrong that it happened, but it is important that Keith not feel more of a victim than he already does.

Luke won't fall asleep unless I'm sitting next to him holding his hand. He tightens and relaxes his grip, then gives up. To-night, after singing the "Moon Song" a few times as written, I changed the words to be about Luke and Daddy and Mama being together at Christmas. Luke was holding my hand but turned away from me in his crib. I don't know how it made him feel. But he fell asleep.

Keith is going to be home at Christmastime. I have no idea why I am so certain, but with Keith in the hospital my resolve is strengthening. It must be so, it will be so. It must and therefore it will. Maybe.

December 5

Tuesday Keith's fever stayed under 102 all day. He felt better but was complaining of pains in his chest. Dr. Davis is begin-ning to think that Keith may have some infection as a result of the surgery.

Wednesday I was jumpy and nervous all day. Keith sounded down on the phone. At five he called to say that his fever was going up again and that he was frightened. The resident thought that he might have pneumonia. I told him not to be scared. When I got off the phone Luke asked, "Why did you tell Daddy not to be scared?"

I gave Luke my undivided attention all evening and put off calling Keith until he was asleep. I called at nine. Keith said he had been put on oxygen. I panicked—too many memories. Sat on a kitchen chair shaking. Called Annie and Robert. Robert came and stayed with Luke; Annie and I went to the hospital. I convinced the security guard that I had a pass to see my husband. He said I could go up for five minutes.

Keith was sick and miserable. Annie went and sat in a chair in the corner and I went to work trying to make Keith comfortable. He started sobbing and said that he was scared and angry. I sponged him down and did what I could to calm him down. Left after about an hour because there was nothing more I could do. Went home with the bubbling of the oxygen machine sounding in my ears. Couldn't unwind. Had a drink and called Karen. Finally fell asleep at one-thirty.

I woke up the next morning with my finger marks imprinted on my upper arms. I had been clutching myself in my sleep. I had dreamt about Keith when I first knew him, in his studio apartment on Fiftieth Street and Tenth Avenue. We took showers together, washed each other's hair. I had dreamt about Keith drying and brushing my hair. I want to care for him.

In the morning Keith's fever was down to 102. He thanked me for last night and said that the general consensus was that he had pneumonia, but not PCP. That evening Annie arrived to sit and I left for the hospital. When I arrived Keith had just taken Tylenol and had his temperature taken: 104. I sponged him down. He was hot, way too hot. I took his temperature: 105. Called the nurse. Told the nurse that she must call Dr. Davis. Another nurse arrived and sponged Keith down with alcohol. About half an hour later they brought in the thermal blanket machine. I went home. I felt as if I were underwater, moving slowly. Everything ached. I wanted to go to sleep.

I woke up with the now familiar feeling of panic. Wanted

the worry to go away, wanted to run away from the telephone. Put off calling Keith until I had given Luke breakfast.

Keith said that his fever was down, and that he felt whatever antibiotic they were giving him was working. He didn't think that his fever would skyrocket again.

That morning I took Luke on an expedition to see the Rockefeller Center Christmas tree and the Saks Christmas windows. We had a really good time. When we got home Luke went right down for a nap, the first in three days.

In the evening Mother took Luke to Brooklyn while I went to see Keith. All my adrenaline was gone. I just felt tired and irritable. Angry at a lost week—a week of worry, then panic, and now exhaustion. Keith, needless to say, looked much better. But he was belching, hiccupping, coughing, and wheezing. All those sounds grated on my nerves. I wanted to go home and get in bed.

December 8

Yesterday Luke and I took Luke's tricycle to the Seminary Park. He can really ride it. I was so proud of him—and so sad that Keith couldn't see him. I thought of how much of Luke's growing up Keith is missing.

Drove Luke to Pat's after his nap and went to the hospital. Now the general consensus is that Keith does have PCP. He had had regular pneumonia and that had made him susceptible to PCP. I walked into his room and he woke up and had a fit of coughing and wheezing. I felt frozen. A wall of exhaustion separated me from the scene. Resentment kept me from touching Keith. True to form, I pretended nothing was bothering me. We had an awful visit.

I can't believe my own reactions. I was jealous that Keith was lying in a bed, cared for. He talked about Christmas plans.

Instead of sounding like fun they sounded like work to me. When Keith said that he had spoken to his parents, who said they had decided to come into the city to "spend a day with their family," I felt like crying. Keith was all gung-ho about how life will be when he gets home, and I felt furious and abused. When am I going to get some rest?

Same old problem: where do you put the anger?

When Luke and I got home that night I knew that if I didn't do something for myself I would end up hurting someone. And knowing me it wouldn't be Keith or Luke, it would be myself.

Annie and Robert took Luke out to breakfast while I went to the gym. Then Luke and I took the bus to St. Margaret's.

We had a picnic lunch on Keith's bed. Keith looks terrible to me. His eyes are puffy and cloudy. He doesn't look all that thin, but his neck is scrawny, as if it would have a hard time supporting his head. His hair is spiky and matted. And he moves so slowly. He seems to be operating in a different time dimension. But Luke didn't seem to notice, or mind if he did. He was thrilled to see his daddy.

I am hoping that they don't let Keith come home until he is stronger—a lot stronger. At the moment I don't feel ready to take care of such a weak person. I think I'll try to be selfish the next few days. Get myself strong for Keith's coming home. I can't stand feeling bitter and angry. I do want him to come home. I think I just don't want to get my hopes up too high. All I can think of are the uncertainties. What if something goes wrong with the Hickman? What if he had a bad reaction to AZT?

Last Wednesday morning Luke and I went up to Macy's to have Luke's hair cut. Luke's first haircut out. I knew when we left the apartment that they were thinking of transferring Keith to another room. We got home and I started washing the windows. It was a beautiful, clear day. The buzzer rang. I looked out the window and there was a long, black limousine. Keith was reentering life on Twenty-first Street in style. Typical of Keith, he'd managed to make all this happen in a matter of hours, talking Dr. Davis into letting him go home instead of transferring him to another room.

Keith amazed me. Just when I was beginning to think of him as an invalid, he regained control. But how he was able to do this in his condition I can't imagine. His eyes are better, but he is extremely weak and tottery. His skin smells like the hospital and disease. And it is transparent, as if made of tissue paper.

Keith is living on a very fragile platform. I feel his fever could reappear at any moment and it could mean anything, anything at all. I have no faith. He looks as though he is very seriously ill. At times he looks scared. And I feel separate from him.

There are times when I wish he wasn't here. Then I think that not having him here would be worse, and I remember how much I wanted him with me only a few days ago. I suppose the times when I don't want him home are times when I really would like him safe, getting stronger somewhere else, so I wouldn't have to worry and feel so responsible for his care. And I could get stronger too, away from him. Then we could meet again.

I know it can't happen that way, but I wish it could. I'm so exhausted that I lose my perspective—I no longer feel any sense of control. I feel that the disease is in control. I will continue to do what I think is right, but there are times when I am so tired I think that by putting myself out to make Keith feel secure and comfortable all I am really doing is making it easier on myself. If anything should happen to Keith, what a comfort it will be to know that I did all I could. I feel guilty at times for having ceased to think that I can make everything all right. Have I given up, given in? Or just realized my limitations?

Tonight I feel as if Keith has left me. That is, the Keith I used to know. I miss the old Keith so much, remember him so vividly. He is not the man asleep in our bed. The man asleep in our bed does not make me feel secure and content. Or inspired and curious. The man in the bedroom is making me feel victimized and angry these days. Our bed seemed more comfortable when he was in the hospital and I could stretch out from side to side. And the worst part of these days is that I can see in Keith's eyes that his worst fear is that I will start to think and feel all the things I just wrote down.

CHRISTMASTIME

We were very social. Saturday the twentieth Keith and I went out together for the first time in almost two months. We went to a dinner that Virginia and Eric gave to celebrate their oldest son's finishing medical school. Driving home down West End Avenue I lost control and started to cry. I felt sorry for myself. I hated everyone at the party for being healthy. I hated Virginia and Eric for having each other and four healthy sons. I hated their security. I was desperately jealous of anyone who felt that his or her life was secure. Angry at them because they seemed to take so much for granted. How dare they? Don't they know it can be taken away at any moment? Their happiness seemed false and superficial.

We got home late and went straight to bed. I lay down and the bed started to reel. I cried and screamed. The anger and sadness seemed endless. Keith got angry. He said I was making things worse. He got dressed to go out. I persuaded him to stay. We talked. Fell asleep at around four.

The next day Rachel came to visit with her baby and Keith went to church. I thought I would feel jealous of Rachel, but I didn't. I guess all the bad feelings got let out the night before. It was nice to have a baby in our apartment. It felt good talking to her about my worries and fears and the everyday difficulties of life. She was sympathetic.

That evening we went to a carol service around the corner at St. Peter's. Luke was dressed in his velvet knickers. I was proud of him. We stayed about half an hour and then went to a friend's Christmas party. Everyone and everything seemed distant and strange, like a foreign country.

Wayne came with us to buy a tree at the lot around the corner. It was good to see Wayne again. We hadn't seen him since before Thanksgiving. On the way home Wayne walked with Luke. He held Luke's hand with his left hand and carried the tree with his right. Keith and I walked slowly, very slowly, behind.

Monday we gave a Christmas party. For some strange reason I had wanted to have a party for family in our house. It backfired. I felt I had put out more than I got back. Went to bed furious.

I saw people being tense about entering our home. It was tension out of concern—it wasn't evil. But it made me furious. How dare they be tense? Here we were working so hard to celebrate our home. Why couldn't they celebrate too?

I think of friends canceling visits because they say they are getting a cold or a virus that they don't want to give to Keith. I think of all the times that's happened, and when I am angry at their tense faces I think, "Really? Was that really why you didn't come?" I feel as though they don't like being around us because we represent things they don't want to face—the fra-

gility of life, disease, the threat of death. But they can't admit
that, maybe not even to themselves. My feelings make me question the sincerity of our friends. And that makes me think I
have lost part of my mind.

It's this feeling that we are different. What we represent to
the world is different from what other families symbolize. I
want a vacation from the difference. Right now everything is
all right in our home. Stop showing me your tense faces.

But pretending everything is all right doesn't work either.
I'm also angered by my family's stiff-upper-lip, push-it-under-
the-carpet approach to difficult, unsettling matters.

Nothing works. Everyone can disappear as far as I am concerned. The parties we've been to as well as the one I gave seem
like so much make-believe. They make me feel like a lost soul
looking longingly at a basket of Easter eggs, each one hollowed
out to contain a perfect little party scene within it—complete
worlds, complex and detailed, encased in way too fragile shells
(though only I know how fragile they are). I want to kick them
away, slam my doors, protect my own. I don't want to think
about anyone else. I want us to live our own lives—just me,
Keith, and Luke.

The week before Christmas Keith bought a new piano. (Keith
had been saying for years that he needed a new piano. We had
left his grand piano in the old apartment, waiting for a buyer.)
We bought it on loan. Spent everything we had in the bank on
the downpayment. It doesn't matter. The money doesn't matter. We could not celebrate Christmas without a piano in the
house.

Keith played Christmas carols. We taught Luke "Jingle Bells."

On Christmas Eve Luke put out a snack for Santa and went
to bed very excited. Keith and I put out the presents and filled

the stockings. Before we went to sleep we stood in the living room and looked around. It looked beautiful. I felt very, very proud of us. Not only had we survived, we had made something good. And Luke's face on Christmas morning confirmed that.

We stayed home and enjoyed.

There was a Christmas once before when Keith and I were completely alone. It must have been five years ago. On Christmas Eve we rented a car, put a small Christmas tree across the back seat, and drove to an inn in Newburyport, Massachusetts. When we arrived we set up the tree in our room and decorated it with the ornaments we had made in England ten years before. We went to midnight mass and came back and made a fire in the fireplace by our bed. In the morning we exchanged presents, then went back to bed and watched the fire. We drove to Plum Island and walked on the beach. Went back to our room and drank brandy and ate canned oysters and cheese and crackers. Joked and philosophized about our life. Felt so blessed, so lucky, and so glad to be away from all pressure.

It was a little like that this Christmas. We were a unit unto ourselves. But this Christmas seemed extraordinarily quiet. I felt as though I were sleepwalking, anesthetized. If I stopped to appreciate I would break down in tears. If I felt my fears I would break the spell. This day was our vacation from the nightmare. We lived the day in stop-time. In the vacuum of those twenty-four hours our home felt blessed and whole. We spoke to our families on the phone and made a special point of calling to thank Dick for the generous check he had given us. It was desperately needed, and Keith and I wanted to make sure he knew how much it meant, how important it was to us. But when I spoke to him I realized the impossibility of conveying to anyone else what things are really like for us. Everyone we spoke to that day seemed to live on a different planet.

January 3

Christmas week our apartment was filled with people every evening. At times that week I felt that this is how I always want to live—in a home filled with friends.

On New Year's Eve we went out for dinner as a family. The waiters hovered around Luke, giving him balloons, confetti, and noisemakers. It was a party.

We came home and sang "Auld Lang Syne" around the piano, then we went to bed together, the three of us curled up in Keith's and my bed. I couldn't help but feel that '87 had to be good (or at least better that '86)—we had ushered it in so well.

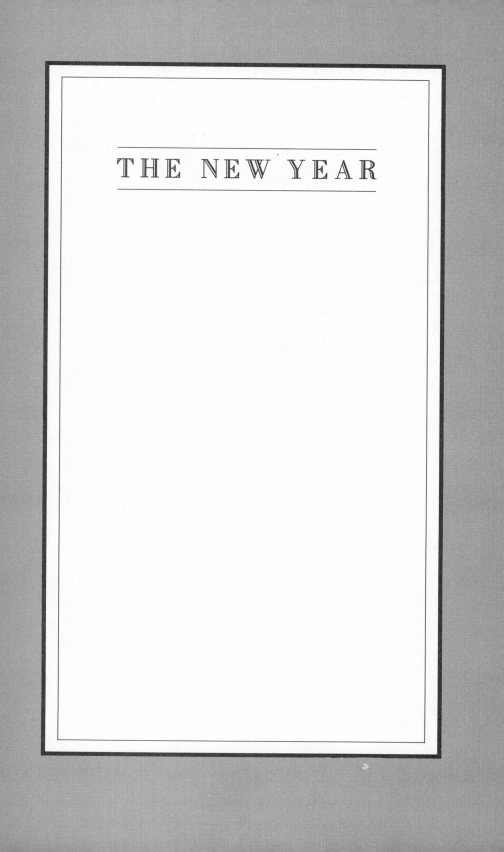

THE NEW YEAR

I was thinking today how life goes on, seems so normal, when Keith is feeling well. We laugh at jokes, we laugh at each other, we delight in Luke. We do the daily chores, sit down to dinner. Keith gives Luke his bath and reads to him before bed. We have one taboo, and that is the future. We don't talk about it, we don't plan for it, we don't have hopes for it, and we don't worry about it (or try not to). We simply live with what is. And, when Keith is here, part of the family, what we have is good. We are aware enough of his disease to know that we must tune in to the present, and that makes things sharper, the nice things better. Living without time. Life is a blessing and we enjoy it, really enjoy it. We know enough to cherish it. We all love each other. Eating pancakes together is a celebration; Christmas was a day in heaven.

Keith takes DHPG three times a week, Monday, Wednesday, and Friday. He prepares it himself—dissolving the powder in water, filling a syringe, injecting the syringe into the saline solution. He hangs the IV bag from the curtain rod over the window next to our bed, then connects the tubing to his catheter. A nurse comes once a week to flush out the catheter and check that everything's all right.

Keith is still driving, at least once a week, to see his therapist, but only when the weather is good. If it is cloudy he says he can't see well enough to drive. He has lost a lot of the peripheral vision in his good eye. He is always turning his head to see what's happening at his side.

Yesterday we drove across town to Altman's and bought a bed for Luke.

One of Luke's Christmas presents, from my mother, was a doctor kit. When we take Keith to his appointments with Dr. Davis, Luke brings it along. When we are called from the waiting room to Dr. Davis's consulting room, Luke grips it tightly and walks very seriously down the hall behind Dr. Davis and his daddy.

January 23

The midwinter doldrums. Stuck in routine. Snowy, icy, and cold outside. Life is quiet and slow, full of procrastinations and stubborn indecisions. Joan, the visiting nurse, comes once a week, on Mondays. Every Monday Joan's arrival puts me in a foul mood. Such an intrusion so early in the morning. I no longer see it as a way of taking the pressure off me. I hate the outside world coming into our home and reminding me that Keith is sick. But Luke loves her coming. He gets out his doctor kit and plays nurse too.

Filled out nursery-school applications for Luke. Finally got a bid on our apartment. Hired a lawyer. Had neighbors of ours from our old apartment, Christian and Lisanne, over for drinks. They don't know Keith is sick. As Luke passed around a plate of cookies Christian asked Keith how he stays so thin.

Luke's bed arrived; we gave his crib to friends. I made curtains for his room. Some nights after Keith or I have read him a story he plays alone in his room and tucks himself in and goes to sleep when he feels ready. He is growing up beautifully.

I went through a period of about five days when I was obsessed with babies. Just plain wanted one. Woke up at night when Luke would call me and thought in my sleepy state that I was going to my two children, that there was a baby with Luke in Luke's room.

I went with Keith to his appointment with Dr. Davis. Dr. Davis plans to stop the DHPG on the 10th of February and start AZT again on the 15th. Keith hasn't taken AZT since his hospital stay when Dr. Davis had taken him off it because he thought Keith was having a bad reaction. He didn't want Keith to start it again until he stopped the DHPG because nobody really knows what the effects of taking the two together are. After he told Keith that he wants him to go back on it now, Keith amazed me by asking him about sperm banks. Was it possible to save his sperm, he wanted to know, as a safeguard against possible damage from AZT? I was touched by his optimism for the future, so impressed with the strength it required for him still to be making plans for the future, still setting his own agenda. But Dr. Davis didn't seem to know what to say. There was a long silence, which Keith finally broke. He said he felt he was losing his masculinity, the power of his sexuality. Dr. Davis looked powerless himself—sympathetic but humbled, almost deflated. He suggested we talk to my obstetrician because he is connected to a hospital with a sperm bank.

I do want Keith's baby, but how can we be thinking about

having another baby now? I want one. And I want Keith's baby. But I know it is impossible now. Nevertheless, I made an appointment with my obstetrician. I know it's unrealistic, but I have to pursue this because it is important to act as if we have options open to us. Especially now, when we feel that doors are closing all around us. Keep as many options open as we can, even if we are just going through the motions.

January 25

Sometime last week Wayne called to say that one of the major networks was doing a piece on "AIDS Buddies" and he was on their list to interview. They want to film a buddy and the person he helps in the AIDS victim's home. Wayne wants them to film him and Keith here. Wayne was calling to ask Keith if he would agree to do it. Keith said he would think about it.

Keith realizes Wayne wants to do it, and he wants to do something for Wayne, but he says it isn't that simple. How do we explain the television cameras to our neighbors? Do we want to have to deal with those issues? And what about Keith becoming public as an AIDS victim? What about Luke?

Keith doesn't want it. He says that we would have to cover up his name on the downstairs buzzer and remove all the labeled tapes of his work from the bookshelves. In other words, erase his identity. Nevertheless, Keith called Wayne and said that he would do it if his anonymity could be respected.

I was confused. Why not come out as an AIDS family? Right now that is what I feel we are. Wouldn't acknowledging it be a healthy thing? I've often thought that Michael Callen has remained strong *because* his ego became so closely tied to the fact that he has AIDS. AIDS and his identity have worked together: he has incorporated AIDS into his self-image. But he's gay and identifies as gay. Keith doesn't. Keith carries a burden of shame.

It seems he will never rise above it. It hurts him and he fights it. He feels like such an anomaly—an AIDS victim who is a heterosexual man with a wife and young child. Part of me wishes he would do the show, be proud to do it, let the neighbors see him on television, let them know what it is like. He cannot and will not. And the decision must be his.

February 1

Last Tuesday Keith went for his appointment with Dr. Christel, the eye doctor. He came home and cried. Dr. Christel said that she continues to be confused by the loss of eyesight in his right eye and says that they have to start thinking of the situation as permanent. My reaction is one of thanks that he still has some sight in his left eye. But I am frightened. It means that if the infection ever returns he doesn't have as much sight to lose. Can't think about it.

Last Wednesday morning Keith said that he didn't feel well. He had been up the whole night coughing. That was nothing new. He has had a sore throat and cough for the past three weeks. But something made him feel that this was different. His temperature was normal at 8 A.M. It was 102 when I left with Luke for play group. It was 104 when we returned at one. Dr. Davis prescribed an antibiotic for Keith to take for two days. If it didn't do the trick he'd admit him to the hospital. Wayne went and got the medicine for us. I helped Keith do his IV of DHPG. He was dizzy and made mistakes and we had to do things over. I wished that I knew how to do it. The old familiar knot in my stomach. Panic and fear. Remote-control actions.

Keith said that he felt short of breath, that he wanted oxygen delivered to the house to get through the night. He called Dr.

Davis, who said that if he needed oxygen he should be in the hospital.

My mother arrived and I packed—down comforter, down jacket, slippers, and toothbrush. Luke said good-bye. A heart-breakingly grownup boy, hiding his fears and confusion. He gave Keith a kiss and said, "I love you with all my heart."

I will never, ever stop hating the drive to St. Margaret's. I will never see St. Margaret's emergency room as anything but a nightmare.

When Keith got settled in bed his fever was down to 100. He had been put in a semi-private room. His roommate was a fortyish man named Don. Don was in the second week of a three-week IV treatment for PCP. He was well enough to be concerned about what sort of person his roommate was, and caring enough to want to get to know Keith and make the best of the situation. I left the hospital glad that Keith was where he could be cared for if his fever peaked again, and glad that he wasn't alone in a room. It was a comfort to me to know there was someone with Keith who could call me if there was a crisis.

That night I missed Keith desperately: everything seemed wrong with him gone. I went to bed but couldn't sleep. When I got up to go to the kitchen or the bathroom I would see Keith in the other rooms—sleeping in the bed or sitting in the rocker in the living room. I slept with the lights on.

I wanted Keith to be home. I remembered his getting up from his nap on "Superbowl Sunday" with rolls of socks stuffed in his longjohns as shoulder pads and a ceramic bowl on his head. Luke put a bowl on his head too. Then they watched the game together.

I wanted to know that he would come home. I thought about last Saturday night when we were discussing Luke's testing us and his need for discipline and structure. I had so much admiration for Keith's ideas, his clear and original thinking. Keith was very emphatic about how we must present ourselves as parents to Luke, let him know that even though we are upset at times, what we are upset about is not his responsibility. Keith is protective of the buffer that separates Luke's childhood world from the nightmare of his parents' world. Whereas I feel my emotions often spill out irrationally onto Luke, Keith interprets our actions for him and explains what is making us upset. I am terrified of being a single parent. And the thought breaks my heart, knowing how good Keith and I are as a team.

When I went to see Keith the morning after he was admitted, Dr. Davis had come and gone. He had had the Hickman catheter taken out (at one in the morning) and had started Keith on an antibiotic IV. He wants to do a workup to see what is causing the fever and cough. He has threatened Keith with a bronchoscopy if his cough doesn't go away, which terrifies Keith (memories of England) and fills me with apprehension because I can't stand to think of Keith alone and in pain. But the antibiotic seems to be working. His fever had gone up to 104 early in the morning, but it didn't go above 102 the rest of the day.

Friday night I was visiting Keith when Dr. Davis was there. No bronchoscopy, thank God, but he is undecided about what treatment to follow in the future. If Keith stops DHPG there is always the possibility that his CMV level will rise, which in Keith's case would probably mean blindness. Keith can't take AZT if he is taking DHPG, because the two together would be too much of an assault on his immune system. Dr. Davis wants to keep Keith in the hospital so they can do a gallein scan and more blood work. I've lost track of what all these tests are supposed to be for.

This seems like a very different hospital stay than the others for two reasons. One is that Keith doesn't seem to be in any immediate danger (famous last words); the other is that he has a roommate.

When I was visiting Keith on Friday, Don had lots of visitors. They looked like fairly hip, attractive, successful New Yorkers. They all left but two, a man and a woman. At one point the woman started crying. She was young and very attractive. After they had left, Don told us that the man was a friend of his from his AIDS support group, and the woman was a workmate who hadn't known he had AIDS. The man had asked Don if the results of his bronchoscopy had come back. When Don said that they were positive, the woman then realized that he has AIDS and started crying.

I was struck by Don's attempts to comfort her. "Don't cry," he kept telling her, "I'll be O.K." I had heard it from Keith so much last year. The incredible beauty of that determination and optimism.

Later Don asked if we wanted to see his KS lesions. He showed us the ones on his legs. They were small, like little purple moles. He said that the ones on his face had been removed by x-ray. I told him that he looked good, that it looked as if his PCP had been caught in time, duck soup compared to what Keith went through in London. Don said that he had lost twenty pounds. He is ordering up food now: eggs from the coffeeshop for breakfast, Chinese food for dinner, milkshakes for snacks.

He said that waiting to get PCP was worse than having it. I got the feeling that he had known his time in the hospital would come and he had planned how to make it a "success"— how to stay in control, manipulate it to his advantage. The self-contained aura of the seriously ill person can be so impressive, so strong. It made me want to pray for him. Keith had been

like Don at the beginning of his hospital stay in November for
his eyes. But he's sick and demoralized now.

There is a room I pass on the way to Keith's room that, like
his room, has an isolation cart outside the doorway and contagion warnings on the door. The two men in the room are very
sick. The man farthest from the door is always asleep. He has a
tube up his nose and tubes in his arms. I've never seen him
awake.

I've never seen the man in the bed nearest the door awake
either. He seems still to be breathing on his own, but he looks
almost comatose—curled up into a fetal position and extremely
thin, emaciated. Out of politeness I try not to look in that
room, but I am haunted by the man nearest the door. A middle-
aged couple sits by his bed. I suppose his parents. They look
out-of-place—midwestern and wholesome. His mother is always
sitting and knitting. She looks determined. The father sits staring out the door. He doesn't seem to notice me or anyone else.
He doesn't look grief-stricken or sad. He just looks puzzled.

That room haunts me. Right now it haunts me more than
Keith's immediate condition. I guess I can't fathom how terrible this disease is.

February 9

The man farthest from the door died last Sunday. That night,
so Don said, a man who had just been diagnosed with AIDS
hanged himself in his hospital bathroom.

The man close to the door died Thursday afternoon. I could
hear his sister (that's who Keith said she was) crying in the
hallway when I went to visit that evening. During my visit

with Keith, Don kept dwelling on the body—why had they left it there for so long? when would they take it away?—and discussing his own funeral. I hate hospitals.

On Friday most of Keith's tests were back. He had PCP again. He was taken off the antibiotic he'd been getting and started on Bactra—once again. Ten days of nausea and feeling poisoned. Keith said that they started the Bactra IV and twenty minutes later he threw up. He's been sick ever since. I went to see him on Saturday and all he could do was doze and throw up. Throw up horrible orange-yellow liquid. Depressing, upsetting visit. Got home and stayed up too late trying to forget it.

Luke woke up at six the next morning. I felt sick from exhaustion. We went down to the Market Square park with his tricycle and he rode and played until it was time to leave. Luke was too tired to walk to the car. He burst into tears, so I picked him up and carried him and the tricycle the two blocks to the car. It was too much. I felt something snap. I burst into tears. Overcome with anger. Screamed at Luke. Was terrified by my anger at Luke and started to sob. Frightened because I couldn't stop crying. Got Luke into his car seat and drove home—both of us in tears. Pure rage. Angry at being alone. Hating everyone who didn't understand, i.e., everybody. Terrified by my weakness. Got home and we both slept and slept.

Feel underwater today. Slow and depressed. At the end of my rope. Going through the motions. Afraid my anger is going to isolate me from the people who can and want to help me.

Keith is extremely nauseous and uncomfortable. When I talk to him on the phone I cannot stand hearing his voice. Every word is an effort for him. I feel like slamming down the receiver. But I miss him desperately. Desperately. And I am sick of having the responsibility of the household and Luke weighing so heavily on me on top of my hurt. I'm sick of AIDS. Sick of hearing about it on the news. (Ads for condoms are a big controversy on the news now. So is how Liberace died). It all seems stupid to me. No more, no less. Stupid and ridiculously naïve.

Keith likens this disease to a rapist—invading completely, without mercy. Attacking unexpectedly and aggressively.

It is impossible to have Keith in the hospital and keep my head above water. Don't know why I thought I could.

February 11

I'm feeling angry and isolated this morning. Wondering when life will be fun again. Angry that nobody has called and said all the right things to make me feel better; nobody has offered to do the things that would make me feel cared for and secure— though what those might be even I don't know. Seems nobody knows what to say, what to do, and I can't help them out. Feeling stuck in a hole. One more terrible February. When will it end? Was thinking that friends don't relax around us anymore. They call to see how we are doing. But they are always watching, never taking part. They don't know how.

I'm getting the feeling that Keith's being so obviously sick now makes people uncomfortable. They don't know how to deal with him in the hospital. So they look to me to tell them it's all right. Or they don't talk about it. Either approach makes me feel isolated.

Sometimes I feel that maybe I am isolating myself, because there are times when I have such feelings of anger toward healthy people. I am desperately jealous of everybody else's life.

*   *   *

Monday night Keith was sleepy—wiped out and groggy. But he looked better to me than he did when he went into the hospital. Something that had been wrong was gone.

He is off Bactra now, and he is no longer feeling so sick. He had a fever of 102 Tuesday night so they are keeping him in the hospital until at least Friday for observation.

I took Luke to see Keith this evening. It was the first time since the PCP that I had seen Keith walking around. He looked weak and frail waiting by the elevators for me to bring Luke up. It was shocking to see him so thin and tottery. He had looked much stronger in bed.

But he did look good to me. I liked looking at him. He is a handsome, striking, interesting-looking man. I felt proud to know him. And I loved feeling those things.

February 15

Keith came home Friday morning. David went to get him. Very white and weak. He had been running a fever between 101 and 102 and having night sweats. Came in and lay down. Luke cut off his hospital bracelet. Keith had just enough energy to supervise my unpacking his things. He went to sleep with his outdoor clothes on.

While Keith was sleeping I was trying to find more drawer space in the dresser next to our bed to put Keith's pajamas. One drawer was filled with the clothes Keith used to wear to the gym. I quietly emptied it. I put the gym clothes in the plastic bag marked "Emergency Services" that they had given him in the hospital. Feeling like a guilty accomplice of fate I stored the bag in the back of Luke's closet.

*   *   *

It doesn't feel cozy to have Keith home at all. It makes me nervous and claustrophobic, as if anxiety and fear have moved into my home to stare me in the face. I can't keep them at bay as I could when Keith was hospitalized. Every time I see Keith in bed my stomach turns over. His face is so thin and drawn that it looks as if his lips wouldn't touch if he closed his mouth. He is coughing a lot. Painful, deep coughs. His skin is scaly and transparent. In between coughing fits he sleeps with his eyes slightly open, with just the whites showing. Diseased. I tell myself that I am always taken aback by how bad Keith looks after a hospital stay, but it doesn't make me feel any better. This is the first hospital stay from which Keith came home still sick. And the doctors can't say what is wrong.

Yesterday Keith's coloring was a little better, but he was nauseous and feverish. He is depressed and angry. Says he doesn't want to die but he can't stand being sick much longer. All I can think about is how tired I am, but when I complained about it to Keith his answer was: "Just think of how much money you'll have for babysitters if I die." That made me furious. It put me in a rage because I felt it was unjust and cruel that suffering and facing death should isolate us from each other instead of bringing us closer. How can I talk about my fears to Keith? How can I ask for his support and sympathy? I can't. When he is sick he and I are living in different worlds. Our concerns are no longer the same. But he's the only person I really want to talk to.

Last night as I was getting into bed at midnight Keith was having a night sweat. Fascinating. I could see the beads of sweat grow and drip. All over—on his forehead, on his arms, on his chest, on his wrists. As if his body were a sponge being wrung out by some mysterious presence. The sweat broke his fever.

Keith is feeling better today. He is coughing less and his fever is down. Last night Luke woke up crying twice. It is bitter cold outside. We are all staying in.

February 16

A morning of confusion and angry inertia. Did Keith want Luke and me to go with him to his appointment at Dr. Davis's? Did I want to go with him? Why couldn't he just say if it was important or not for us to take him? Was it important? On and on. In the end we took him. Luke was scattered, I was angry. Dr. Davis recommended Keith start taking AZT again at a full dose: two pills every four hours.

I was withdrawn on the drive home—furious that Keith was so self-involved, so lost in his own thoughts. I lost my temper. We fought.

How can I talk to him about my fears? How can I listen to his? Every time he approaches the subject of death I close up; come up with platitudes like "I don't want you to die. There is still hope." No help at all. My fear and anger become worse because I don't speak them—they become a horrible burden. Then Keith becomes a burden because he represents all the fears. Life is harder with him home. The housework and caring for Luke grate on my nerves because Keith is home and I am wondering why he isn't helping out (the answer is obvious). Support from family and friends isn't as forthcoming when Keith is home. Keith is home but he isn't a friend or comrade. I have a husband but I don't.

Keith is so sensitive to anything that can be interpreted as pushing him out, excluding him from his home life, reminding him that he isn't as productive a member of the household as he once was, that many of the things I say and do are misinterpreted. Our frustrations are volatile, incendiary. We take out all our anger on each other.

There are moments when Luke's presence seems to make things worse. As if his abundance of energy and enthusiasm only accentuate Keith's dwindling reserves, cruelly pointing up the fact that Keith can't father in a hands-on way. But the other night, when Keith didn't feel well enough to read Luke his bedtime stories, Luke went and got his book, very cheerfully climbed in bed next to Keith, and "read" *Madeline* to him.

We got home from Dr. Davis's and fought and cried. Poor Luke fell asleep on the living-room floor while we muddled through our feelings in the bedroom. Finally we cried together. Crying felt so good. Peculiar state of affairs when crying becomes a treat, a luxury, a tonic. Soothing.

After crying out the tension of the last two and a half weeks I thought of how schizophrenic my life is. When Keith is in the hospital I steel myself for living alone. Without consciously realizing it I am practicing. While making dinner, bathing Luke, putting Luke to bed, sleeping alone, part of me is always thinking, Is this what it will be like? Can I do this? Yes, maybe I can. Then Keith comes home and my allegiances shift. Part of me feels interrupted; my pattern, my plan, my defenses seem crazy, irrelevant. Becoming Keith's comrade again is painful. It means accepting the fact that I missed him, will miss him horribly. That I hated his being in the hospital, that I hate his being sick. That I hate him for handling his suffering so bravely when I don't know if I can. Being close to Keith means facing so much anger and pain. Screaming rage and tears form the bridge from me to him.

I came home from taking Luke out and heard Keith on the phone. I heard him say, "This is it." And he hung up. I asked who he was talking to. He said he was talking to his therapist's answering machine. He said he didn't want to talk to his therapist anymore. That he didn't help. He didn't understand. I pointed out that he had been helpful in the past. Keith said that was irrelevant now. He said he had told his therapist about how we used to make love outdoors in the woods the first summer we were together. He smiled and said, "I just want to think about that now."

Friday night when Keith was too weak to put Luke to bed, Luke came into our bedroom and put his blanket over Keith. He carefully straightened it and tucked it around Keith. "Get cozy, Daddy."

March 1

The week of February 16 to 21 was a nightmare. For the first time I thought that if this is how Keith's life is going to be, if he has to suffer this much, then I would rather it ended. There is no point to this kind of suffering. Keith's fevers never went away; they got worse. He followed a pattern of being normal in the morning, then by early afternoon a cycle would start: first he would get a chill, then his fever would climb, then he would break out in a sweat, then the fever would break.

Monday through Wednesday weren't so bad. But by Thursday it was scary. His chills were so bad they shook the bed. Nausea came with the fever. His fevers were hovering around 104. He threw up during the chills. The sweats were drenching. He was getting thinner and more drawn (dehydrated) every day.

Luke was getting concerned and confused. He would check the bedroom before we went out and as soon as we came home. By Friday I was frightened by how exhausted I felt. We didn't call Dr. Davis. We were afraid he would put Keith back in the hospital. In retrospect it seems crazy to me that we didn't call him. But we were scared. It was as if we felt that Keith was too sick to go to the hospital, that what was going to happen should happen at home. Keith had an appointment to see Dr. Davis Saturday, so we waited until then.

Saturday Dr. Davis said that Keith was experiencing a reaction to AZT. The dose he's been taking was too strong for him. He should stop taking it until the following Wednesday and then start up again, taking half of what he had been taking. He gave Keith a prescription for acetaminophen, which he said would "trick" Keith's body into acting as if there were no fever. We left Dr. Davis's office reassured and relieved. We all slept well that night.

Sunday I took Luke down to the Market Square park with Marianne and Jacob. It was a beautiful warm day. When we got home Keith was on the phone with Dr. Christel. He was saying that he was losing the sight in his good eye. He was going blind. Horrifying. Horror is the only word that fits. Keith said that if he was going blind he would want to kill himself. I nodded my head. I could only agree with him—I supposed I would feel the same way if I were in his situation. But I couldn't think about it then. Why jump to conclusions before Dr. Christel saw Keith in the morning? For the first time in over a year, I took one of Keith's tranquilizers. His fever was hovering around 102. He would start getting chills and then take an acetaminophen pill to break the fever's cycle.

Luke and I took Keith to Dr. Christel's. I didn't feel particularly anxious or scared. I felt anesthetized to those feelings, as if sleepwalking. But I did feel admiration for Keith. For his courage. He could have gotten in bed, hid under the covers, and waited to die. But here was Keith, dragging himself to the doctor, dealing with reality, looking for solutions, confronting the uncertainties and ambiguities of his situation. I guess hiding under the covers is what I want to do.

Dr. Davis was out of town so his replacement and Dr. Christel decided that Keith should go into the hospital immediately, have a Hickman put in, and start DHPG again. They would put the catheter in as soon as the surgeon could do it. Luke and I walked Keith across the street to St. Margarget's emergency room and left him. Luke was upset that Keith wasn't coming home with us. We went to the Third Avenue Lamston's and bought some new toys. Went home and played with them and then slept.

The next morning they put in the catheter with no problems. I hate it. It is on his left side this time, the side next to me in our bed, the shoulder I like to lie on.

For the first three days in the hospital, Keith took his acetaminophen every eight hours without telling the doctors or nurses. He was terrified that, if the knew about his fevers, they would start the inevitable cycle of tests and treatment again. He was only concerned with getting medication to save what was left of his sight. He figured if he could keep his fever down they would leave him alone, at least until Dr. Davis came back on Thursday night.

Keith has been put on the oncology floor in the most claustrophobic room imaginable. The room is a narrow rectangle: two beds foot to foot. There is one window across from the bed that you practically bump into when you walk in the door. From Keith's bed you can't see it. His bed is next to the bathroom door, so close that his roommate couldn't get into the bathroom with his IV pole (he is being treated for CMV) until I moved Keith's bed closer to the opposite wall. Keith is stuck in a corner, with no natural light. You can't tell if it's day or night in that room. Keith says he is confused about what time it is, what day it is. He leaves the TV on to act as an anchor, some connection to the outside world.

Wednesday Dr. Christel said that Keith's left eye had improved enormously. She wanted to increase the dosage of DHPG because it was obviously working well. But in the afternoon his blood work came back. He was severely anemic and his white count was less than one. They decided to give him a day off from DHPG because it was too dangerous with his white count so low. When I arrived in the evening he was having a blood transfusion.

Thursday he felt better and looked better, less skeletal and drawn. But he had a fever and was desperately weak. The infectious-disease doctors came to see him and told him to get rid of the flowers in his room (a pot of jonquils I had brought) and to stop drinking the bottle of Evian water Keith liked to keep by his bed. His white count was so low that the microorganisms in the earth around the flowers and in the water were dangerous to him. Keith and I couldn't believe that bottled water could be a serious threat—or earth for that matter. As Keith said, "What if you live in the country?" I think the doctors are going a little crazy trying to keep him germ free. But we do what they say because we're afraid not to. Dr. Davis saw him that night. He said he was ordering some antibiotics to try to get whatever was causing the fevers.

Friday morning Keith was so desperately weak it hurt me to watch him move. I arrived to find him sleeping with the TV on. I woke him up, but his eyes would close if there was a lull in our conversation. He said that a group of doctors had come to his room with Dr. Christel and told him he had to choose between longevity (AZT) and his eyesight (DHPG). Keith said he wanted to save his eyesight at all costs. Hard for me to hear—especially since I know how little good the DHPG can do now that Keith has already lost so much of his vision. Keith said to me that he felt he had control over his will to live, hence his longevity, but no control over the CMV and his eyes. I was amazed and relieved he felt he still had any control. Keith continues to rally at points where I know I would give up if I were he. I admire him so much for that.

Friday evening Keith was even weaker. His fever was down but he was having terrible sweats. He said they changed his bed five times Thursday night. Dr. Davis had come to see him and said that his white count had dropped even further, from .8 to .7. Keith said he had asked Dr. Davis if this was it. Was his body stopping, breaking down completely? Dr. Davis asked Keith if he thought it was. Keith said no. Then Dr. Davis asked Keith what he would like him to do if it was. Keith said to get him out of the hospital. Get him home.

March 8

All last week it was cloudless and sunny outside. I walked to the hospital every evening, as the sun was going down. I talked to myself as I walked. I would go through in my mind everything that had happened that day: what Luke had done, what Keith had said on the phone, what I had done. Usually I would walk a block or two out of my way to give myself more time. When I found myself near St. Margaret's I would panic. Scared of going inside. Scared of what was waiting inside for me.

One morning I left Luke with Annie. I saw Keith in the hospital, then drove to our old apartment. Keith's piano is the only thing left there. New windows were about to be put in and his piano needed to be wrapped up, protected from the workers and the cold. I covered it with an old sheet. I ripped pages out of a notebook and wrote, "Please do not touch," "Please treat with care." I put the papers on the piano, looked at them, and collapsed. Good-bye. It is over. Please protect. Oh God, please protect.

I lay on my stomach and held the floor with my hands. I rolled over and looked at the ceiling. I followed its edges with my eyes, tracing where it met the walls. I got up and walked into the bedroom, sobbing, holding my stomach. It is gone. Life has left these walls. Keith's piano is standing here cold. I looked out the window and felt the pain of loss move from my burning eyes and convulsing throat to my chest and shoulders. I can carry it there. I know I can carry it there. And as long as it burns I will be all right. If I can feel it burning I can go on. If I feel I am carrying the memories I will be all right. I left the door unlocked so the workers could get in.

Keith's white count began to go up, but he was still having fevers (although nothing above 103) and night sweats. On Monday afternoon he called me. He said that he was being put on TPN (nutritional IV feeding) that was to continue for twelve hours a day at home. He was sobbing. He said he had no one to talk to—he felt scared and alone. Said he was having terrible nightmares. I said that I would ask Susan to come to the hospital tomorrow morning for a joint therapy session. Keith said he thought that would be a good idea.

When I went to visit that evening I made him as comfortable as I could and told him he was not alone, he was going to go home. As I was getting ready to leave he said that he didn't think he wanted to have a therapy session in the hospital.

He wants to talk and then he doesn't. Fear and anger and remorse about dying come and go. I feel the same way. When my fear and grief hit it is real: I know Keith's death is coming. Then I see Keith and he is alive. Or I am taking Luke to the grocery store or putting him to bed and I wonder how I could have thought the things I did. Those thoughts/feelings seem to have no place in the daily world. I start to wonder if I felt them in a dream. Did I really cry about Keith's death last night? I can't believe my thoughts are real. My grief and fears come and go, like chills on a warm day. When they are gone I wonder if they really happened. And sometimes I feel guilty and worry that if I think about Keith's dying and and make attempts to "prepare" for it I am hastening his death. Taking away support for his living. A saboteur. But at night all my tears come. My spirits plummet with the light. My stomach becomes hollow. These feelings are too overpowering to be imagined or fabricated. Or denied.

I feel the need to talk to Dr. Davis. I feel panicked and angry about Keith's situation. Keith is beginning to talk about his own death but he is being more and more isolated, both by the ambiguities of his illness and its seriousness. The ambiguities create a vacuum of confusion and despair because no one can say exactly what is wrong. And the seriousness of his disease means that the hospital staff treat him like a terminally ill person. They don't talk to him about anything but the most superficial concerns; they isolate him. They obviously are uncomfortable about being around someone that sick.

I am terrified that what is left of Keith's health will deteriorate quickly—a snowball effect in which one thing leads to another and he cannot ever come home. I tell myself that if that happens I will carry him home on my shoulders.

The morgue at St. Margaret's is in the basement. They have a poinsettia left over from Christmas in the window. The window is under some sidewalk grating on Seventeenth Street, and when it is open I can see the saws and blood in the sink. I know where it is because one night Luke was standing on the grating and asked to be carried, so I bent down to pick him up and saw it. That happened when Keith was in the hospital in January, but the morgue is really haunting me now.

I can no longer do this alone. I need more help. The circle of support is too small. I cannot sit with the parents of Luke's friends in the playground and answer the question "How are you?"—listen to them chat about their lives and have them ask innocently about mine. I will lose my mind.

Worse than keeping the secret is not knowing how they would respond. So I decided to test the waters by calling my cousins Charlie and Donna-Maria, who have a daughter Luke plays with. I guess part of me felt that they were safe. They had to be accepting, they were family.

Donna-Maria was accepting. I suppose she was sympathetic. I couldn't tell. All I felt was that I was talking to someone on another planet, someone who spoke a different language. My words came out but they didn't say what I felt, didn't seem to explain anything—words without a context.

Then I called Jacob's mother, Marianne. I said, "Keith has AIDS," and she burst into tears. She told me about a friend of hers who had died. She talked about how Jacob had responded to his death, how she had told him. I liked her openness. In a funny way it was soothing. But it also frightened me.

I must get my nerve up to talk to Dr. Davis.

Wednesday evening I arrived at the hospital and Keith was sitting up in a chair in his room crying. Miserable. He said that it was very important to him that I learn to administer the TPN as soon as possible. He was obsessed with my learning immediately. Said if I learned then he could go home. I knew that wasn't true. But I said I would be back the next morning for a lesson.

He is so terrified of being abandoned.

Early the next morning Keith called to say that Dr. Davis had been in and told him that he had tuberculosis. Keith sounded defeated by the news, but my reaction was relief. I know this is ludicrous, but at least something has a name. Now he has something with a name, hence a set course of treatment to follow. A path to getting better.

I took Luke up to Pat, who was going to take him to work with her, and then I went to the hospital for my first TPN lesson. I loved it. It made me feel involved and useful. There was something soothing about the fact that there was an important, practical part of Keith's medical care that I could do myself. It will take me a while to learn all the steps, but once I learn it will be another way we can be independent of the doctors and nurses who seem to be taking over our lives now. We desperately want to feel in some kind of control.

Keith fell asleep halfway through the lesson. Devastatingly weak. He is gaining weight (they started the TPN on Tuesday) but it is a funny kind of weight gain. He has no muscle tone and his skin is white and flaky. A body full of chemicals, fed on chemicals.

When I went back that evening, Keith had been moved into a private room. There was space, and with it huge psychological relief. And Keith was a little stronger. When I arrived he was ending a two-hour visit with his cousin. He was tired, but not wiped out. I decided to bring Luke the next evening

Luke has been very concerned about his daddy. The evening that Keith went into the hospital Luke took out the plastic knives that he uses for Play-doh and started attacking my chest. I asked him if he thought that is what they were doing to Daddy in the hospital. I explained about the catheter in Keith's chest. We need to explain it all to him.

Luke asked why Daddy was in the hospital. Why does he need the nurses to take care of him? I tell him now that Daddy has a virus in his blood. It makes him very sick—too sick to take care of himself. There are things in the hospital he needs that we don't have at home.

One night last week Luke woke up at three-thirty and came into our bedroom. He said that he wanted to play. He was sort of sleepwalking, not really awake. I told him it was still night-time and guided him back to his bed. When I got him back into his bed I saw that he had pulled the curtains on his windows back, as I do in the morning. I asked him about it. He said, "I pulled my curtains back so I could see the white building and then Daddy could see it too."

For a couple of nights last week Luke slept with his arms around the picture of himself and Keith sitting by the river in Germantown. I also heard him trying to make retching sounds by putting his fingers down his throat—like his Daddy throwing up. When I asked if he was all right he smiled. Said he was all right, and to leave him alone.

Luke was anxious to go to the hospital Friday night. We walked as far as Sixth Avenue before we got in a cab. As I pushed Luke in the stroller he called out, "Yuuuuhooo, Daddy, we're coming."

When we walked into Keith's room Luke gave Keith an enormous, solemn hug. He got in bed with Keith and watched TV, made the bed go up and down, and recited nursery rhymes. Then he became very quiet and serious. I asked him if he would like to be alone with Daddy. Keith said, "Maybe Mommy has to go to the bathroom." Luke said yes, he would like that.

Looked at me and said, "Go." I went into the bathroom and closed the door. Glued my ear to the door but couldn't hear. Later when we were leaving there were no tears. Luke just looked at Keith and said, "See you later, alligator."

Tomorrow I have an appointment to talk to Dr. Davis. I am very nervous. I don't know if I am scared of what he will tell me or scared that I won't be able to explain my concerns and convictions. I want Keith to die at home—absolutely, no doubts or ifs. I feel I would never recover if Keith died in the hospital. But I am not sure I can manage it. And how do I explain how important that is to me when everything in me is screaming that I don't want Keith to die?

I want Luke to see that, despite the pain and anguish, death is organic and natural, a part of life. That you care for the dying—respect the dying. Please may he remember the caring. If he has to lose his daddy, at least let him see his parents loving each other, caring for each other. Caring for him. Dying with due respect for life.

I pray for the strength to make it so. In this home. I think I can do it. I think maybe the strength to do it has to do with finding the power of unconditional love.

March 10

Dr. Davis confirmed all my fears and in his take-charge way was a step ahead of me in plans. Luckily we were in agreement. Reassurance of a kind. He wants to put Keith in the hospice program at St. Margaret's: "Home care for the terminally ill with the least amount of home disruption."

I walked home. It was getting cold and windy and cloudy and damp. Weird after two days of spring weather. I didn't

understand how my feet could be touching the ground, walking—I didn't feel as though I were standing on the ground. My
perspective and perception of distance had changed. Everything
looked foreign to me. I was walking through a movie set. This
wasn't my home neighborhood anymore. This was where my
husband was going to die. Where life as I knew it was going
to end. I stared at our apartment building, but turned down
the wrong street.

Luke was hyper, exhausted, crying, and miserable when I got
home. He had been terrified of my going to see Dr. Davis.
Scared I wouldn't come back. I calmed him down and he fell
asleep on his bedroom floor.

I went into the living room and sobbed. The pain: tangible,
physical pain in my bones. I remembered it from London; it
was familiar. But this time I knew it was only the beginning
of the pain I would be feeling. I cannot conceive of finding the
strength to get through this. But I know I will. What I don't
know is how I will survive Keith's being gone—how I will
survive the pain of having to go on without him. Even though
the inevitability of his dying has become more tangible it is
still inconceivable to me.

Knowing that Keith is going to die makes it easier to plan,
easier to act on what were only nighttime fears and ambiguous terrors. Finally my nightmares are becoming a reality, but
their reality is a twilight zone where I wander about, flighty
and jumpy, scared and hurting. My only anchors are the smell
of Keith's skin and the feeling of Luke in my arms. My
teeth chatter and my eyes burn when I think that Keith will
be gone.

Dr. Davis had said that he would talk to Keith about hospice
in the morning: tell him he would be coming home to die. It
hurts to think of Keith scared and alone in his hospital room.
But as of ten tonight, Dr. Davis hadn't shown up.

*   *   *

I went to see Keith this morning and he still had not been told.
But he is ready. We talked about his death without mentioning
the word. I cried. I lay down on Keith's bed with my head on
his shoulder. I listened to him sleep. I dozed. I could hear the
nurses tiptoe around the bed trying not to disturb us.

On the way home I thought of the paragraph from *Anatomy
of an Illness,* the book by Norman Cousins I read last spring.
"Death is not the ultimate tragedy of life. The ultimate tragedy
is depersonalization—dying in an alien and sterile area, separated from the spiritual nourishment that comes from being
able to reach out to a loving hand, separated from a desire to
experience the things that make life worth living, separated from
hope."

But how can you not be separated from hope when you are
dying? I keep thinking that being separated from hope is a
terrible, terrible thing.

I took Luke to see Keith tonight. It was late, Luke and I were
tired. I had forgotten Luke's special blanket. Luke gave Keith
a heartfelt hello and many good-bye kisses, but the visit was
hard on him. It wasn't special; he had been in the room before.
And he was upset by how sick Keith is. He sees that his daddy
has changed. Keith was nauseous. He threw up. Luke wanted
to go home.

When we got home we had a picnic supper of noodles in
front of the TV. Unfortunately the show we were watching unexpectedly had a scene of a man in bed, with a nurse and family
standing around. The man retched and spit up. Luke started
screaming, "Change the channel, go to another channel."

*　*　*

I called the Haileys. We'd been out of touch for months, but I knew they would want to know how serious Keith's situation is now. Their response was comforting. Virginia said that she had finished her exams, and her time was ours.

Now Virginia sits with Keith in the hospital for hours. She calls me and asks what she can do. Her thinking is clear and practical, sympathetic and very caring. A comfort. I was thinking last night, or rather trying not to think, that perhaps some things do come full circle. I met Keith babysitting for Virginia and Eric's children. They were our introduction. Now they are helping with our parting.

Last night Luke put Keith's old hospital bracelet on Dolly, tucked a hypodermic syringe from his doctor kit under her arm, wrapped her in a cloth diaper, and said that he was taking care of her. When I changed his diaper at 2 A.M., Dolly's blanket and "medicine" had been kicked all over the bed. When Luke got out of bed at 8:30 this morning they were all back in place.

This morning Luke told me that when I go to visit Keith in the hospital he is afraid that I will "disappear." He is terrified of my leaving him like Keith. Tonight Luke added Zebra to the scenario in his bed. Zebra is tucked in next to Dolly. She's Dolly's mother, Luke says; Paddington is Dolly's father. I asked him if Dolly's father was sick or well. He said well. When I said that I understood that it was hard to have a sick daddy, he said that he wants Daddy to be well "so much." Sometimes I think that now may be the time to tell him that Daddy isn't going to get well.

SPRING

L arry, Eric, and I brought Keith home over a week ago, Saturday night the 14th. Keith had had a fever the previous night, Friday, so Dr. Davis wanted to keep him in the hospital the next day to watch him. He said he would be there Saturday evening to make the decision about whether or not to discharge him. Larry, Eric, and I were there waiting when Dr. Davis arrived. He said that Keith could go home. Weak and frail. White, flaky skin. His breath smelling foul; heavy with disease and chemicals. I was amazed that Keith made it in the front door. A virtually blind, miserable skeleton.

The first three days at home Keith had terrible anxiety attacks. He shook and cried. He would sit up in bed, his arms extended in front of him, and shake and cry out in rage and frustration. Then he would collapse in tears. Someone had to be with him all the time: to hold his hand, to tell him he wasn't alone, to tell him where he was. The Haileys' had bought a stereo for the bedroom. Keith wanted the radio on at all times. At night he had hallucinations. Once I came to bed and he asked me if he was in the right corner. Was he in the right place? Where were the other children? Who was I? As if he thought he was a child again in the polio hospital.

We got him some tranquilizers and sleeping pills. Gradually there were some hours at a stretch when he was calm, asleep.

Eric set up a buzzer for Keith to ring if he needs me. It is like a makeshift doorbell. The button Keith pushes lies next to his hand in bed and the bell that rings sits on the floor in the hall outside our bedroom. Its ring is loud and intrusive. I hear it constantly, when Keith rings it and when he doesn't. I always imagine I hear it when I am taking a shower at night—I run out of the shower with shampoo in my hair only to find Keith sleeping.

Keith's extreme anxiety gradually left. But he stayed miserable, hating the days and hating the nights. The TPN started the Monday after he came home. DHPG is every other day, immediately following the TPN. Supplies were delivered over the weekend—carton after carton filled with bags and bottles and tubes and syringes. Bags of medicine have taken over the refrigerator. Cartons line the hall. Our home has been invaded by Keith's medicine.

Nurses came to make sure I knew how to administer the TPN and DHPG. I hate them. I hate having them in our home. Keith gets anxious and starts to shake while they are here. I hate it when they talk to me in the kitchen as if Keith weren't involved in this: "You're in for a long haul." "I hate to tell you, but these pills he is taking [$200 worth, and that's from a drugstore that sells to AIDS patients at cost] don't do anything." Asking, "How is your son handling this?" while Luke is playing on the floor right next to us.

The visiting nurse comes at eight in the morning. That is when Keith's twelve hours on the TPN IV are over. Keith feels awful when the TPN finishes, dizzy and disoriented. Once he told the visiting nurse that he can't sleep at night—that he is restless and gets confused, then hallucinates. The nurses see it as a physical symptom: they think CMV may be attacking his brain. They don't say that out loud, of course, but every morning they ask Keith to count backward by sevens from ninety-eight. I assume his hallucinations and confusion are from his extreme anxiety, a part of his trying to make peace.

I'm feeling completely overwhelmed. Luke needs to be taken out or supervised when I do the medicine. And, if the nurses are here, Luke needs extra attention; he is demanding and clingy. Keith needs someone with him always. If I want any time for myself, I have to organize two sitters—one for Keith and one for Luke.

When I go out I take a beeper with me. Anyone staying with Keith has instructions on how to beep me. The phone number is over every phone in the apartment. Away from Keith I test it constantly. In the grocery store I push Luke's stroller with one hand, test my beeper with the other.

All my time is spent organizing and administering. No time for Keith, no time to be alone with him. My romantic notions of curling up with Keith at night, being close to him, have evaporated. He's too anxious to talk, or else in a drugged sleep. I'm too exhausted and resentful to think about the days, about what is happening. People here in the morning, people here in the evening. Never alone. Always exhausted. But some days, when Keith is asleep and Luke is taking his nap, everything gets blissfully peaceful and quiet for a while. Like a house with a sleeping newborn in it.

At night when Luke's asleep, before I get in bed with Keith, I obsess about plans. Who is coming tomorrow? Who can bring groceries? What do we need? Friends have given their time: Arlene has committed to Monday mornings, Polly to Wednesdays, Robert various afternoons. Wayne is away in California for the next couple of weeks. Some evenings Annie comes to watch Luke while I do Keith's medicine, and sometimes Pat, Larry, and Brandon take Luke out to dinner. Virginia is a wonderful constant.

I go over and over the schedule in my head, hating it all but trying to make peace with it, get to know it, convince myself that yes, this is a life, this could go on forever. Arlene is good with Keith: I can go out with Luke. Luke likes playing with Polly: I will stay with Keith. Virginia is bliss because I can play it by ear; she is great with both Keith and Luke. I wonder if I should call the people coming the next day—will they remember? I take my beeper out of my bag and check it—is it working?

And then I get in bed with Keith and we both cry. And for a few minutes everything is all right. In a strange way it feels wonderful. Deep, deep sobs. We are sharing our pain, crying over the past year and a half, crying over the lost future. Doing it together, dissolving months of aloneness. Sharing the pain of the unspeakable fact: Keith is going to die. Keith doesn't want to die. I don't want him to die. We are both scared; we both don't want it to happen. We don't want to be separated. We cry and cry and are united again.

One night while I was checking the TPN tubing Keith and I heard Luke talking to himself in his bed. "Av-eh," he said, "Av-eh-don . . . Uh-huh, Luke *Avedon*. We had never heard him say his last name before. Keith smiled. I got teary.

I don't want it to hurt so much. I say to Keith, "You will see Luke grow up, I know it." Keith looks at me and says, "I know I will."

But Keith stares. Keith lies in bed and stares. Staring and staring. Staring straight ahead even though his eyes can hardly see. I cannot fathom what he is staring at, what makes him need to lie with his eyes wide open. Staring straight ahead for hours.

One afternoon Arlene arrived while Keith was sleeping. She waited in the living room while I went in to Keith. I sat with him until he woke up. He opened his eyes and said, "Who is in the apartment?" He senses everything.

Yesterday, when Keith had been home a week, I knew that things were as good as they were going to get. I had the house organized and clean. Helpers and babysitters were available and around. We had found a nurse's aide to come three days a week, ten to one, to bathe and shave Keith. But Keith and I are so miserable. We aren't talking much. On the days a nurse comes, I can't make it to noon without bursting into tears. On Keith's good days he is resigned and withdrawn. And at special moments, like Luke sitting on Keith's lap in the rocker watching *Sesame Street,* our hearts break.

And I do not know myself. I am so thin. I feel brittle and hard. I am eating but wasting away, as if I am being pulled into a different dimension along with Keith. Do I want to go too?

Keith says that he isn't afraid of dying but he is afraid of two things: going back into the hospital and the disease destroying

him little by little, over a long period of time. I can only re-
assure him that he will not go back into the hospital. But the
disease will go on for a while, I know. Joan, the nurse, speaks
to me in terms of "When you get to the final month or two."

March 26

Our fears and sadness we share now. Everything else is an intrusion. And I hate it. We hate it. Hate the nurses, the para-
phernalia of caretaking. Now we are together—why can't Keith
and I do it alone? I don't want the rhythms of our household
broken by all these outsiders. I want things peaceful. When
Keith dies I want to wake Luke in the morning: I want to close
Keith's and my bedroom door and then walk into Luke's room
to tell him. I want the drama of Keith's dying to remain within
these walls, within our family. In our home as we love it, not
a hospital outpost. The three of us. Keith made this home. I
want him to be proud of it, of himself, of us.

Last Tuesday morning a wheelchair was delivered and Victor
(the nurse's aide) took Keith out. I was off doing errands with
Luke. When I got home Keith was on the phone to Virginia.
In tears. He was saying that his situation was too cruel: it was
so beautiful out but it was no longer his world. He doesn't
belong here anymore.

When he hung up the phone he said he had told Virginia
that he wanted to die and Virginia had said that if he really
wanted to she would help. I gave him a hug to let him know I
would support him in whatever he wanted to do, but I didn't
really absorb what he was saying. How could I?

Susan came for a session here at home with Keith and me.

We sat in the living room in our rocking chairs. Again I listened to Keith say that he wanted it to end. We talked about it, and with Susan there to guide us—to neutralize the charge of the conversation—what had been unspeakable, unthinkable, became a normal option, which could be discussed. More than an option, a viable alternative.

"Look at Elizabeth, Susan," Keith said. "Look how exhausted she is. I am destroying my family." I bit my lip to keep from protesting; I simply listened. I realized that one reason Keith wants to die quickly is for me, for Luke. He sees it as a way of helping us out of an impossible situation. As we talked, it became obvious to me that to Keith it was the only way he had to preserve his dignity. And his self-respect. A way of making his dying an affirmation of his life.

And because of that it seemed right. It is the only thing that has happened in a very long time that has enabled me to draw upon the courage of my convictions.

We talked about when. Keith said soon, perhaps next Tuesday.

Wednesday morning while Luke was at the playground with friends, Virginia, Keith, and I talked and made plans. Frighteningly mundane facts to be learned: Does suicide cancel Keith's life-insurance benefit? How do we keep the visiting nurses from being suspicious? How can we be sure that Dr. Davis will write "natural causes" on the death certificate? What must we do so that if Keith's death looks suspicious I will not be implicated. What drug will work?

Virginia left the room to make phone calls. Keith and I held each other. We sobbed. I cannot believe that the earth will go on spinning, that the sun will come up and go down after Keith is gone. I cannot really believe that Keith will ever be gone. And yet I am planning his death with him. Crying on his shoulder, nestling in his arms. Our tears are warm. We acknowledge our final joint effort. In some ways it feels like planning for the birth of Luke.

After we talked and cried and cried and talked, I took Keith out for a walk in the wheelchair. We went to the Seminary Park. It was cloudless, warm, and still. We floated. I parked the wheelchair on a pathway and helped Keith around to the far side of an old stone building. We sat on the ground and leaned on the warm stones. We held each other. Separate from the rest of the world; totally tuned in to each other. Floating and aware; self-contained and blissfully happy. We felt blessed. The world seemed magical. We had a place in it again. We were no longer trapped.

The rest of the day was spent making phone calls. A strange adrenaline rush. Excited and determined. Making lists and feeling free.

Keith and I made an appointment to speak to Dr. Davis on Saturday. We're hoping to get Dr. Davis's support. But we have a backup plan in case we don't.

Today we came down to the reality of the blood man at seven-thirty; Joan, the nurse, at eight; Victor, the nurse's aide, at ten. I didn't get to talk to Keith all morning. He had had bad dreams. I was overtired. By afternoon I was terrified and jumpy. By evening I was just plain terrified. Sick to my stomach. Annie came to help and served Keith and me dinner in bed. After Luke had been put to bed I lay in bed holding my churning stomach. The room began to spin when I saw the Hemlock Society's book on my bedside table.

I am sitting in the kitchen now, trying to think it all through. I know that this dread and fear have to be experienced and worked through. I am terrified of Keith's leaving this earth. Terrified of how great the pain of missing him will be. Terrified of being alone. Every cell in my body wants my family intact. And I am planning my husband's death.

"Tell Luke I didn't want to die. I didn't want to leave him. Be sure and tell him I didn't want to die. He will be angry at me for dying when he is older. I can't stand to think of him being angry at me, but he will be. Tell him I didn't want to die."

March 28

Last night, at my request, Rachel came with baby Aaron to visit so that we could tell her our plans. I wanted her to know. Keith wants me to have someone with me. He is concerned that I have some support, some help. He thinks it might be best if Eric was here because he is a psychiatrist; he could offer the most help if, God forbid, anything went wrong. I feel that if I decide that I do want someone with me (but I don't think I will) I would want it to be someone in my family.

Dead silence in the living room when Keith and I told Rachel. Then she started crying. Said that she didn't want Keith to die. That she couldn't imagine him gone. But that she understood our wishes. She said that she admired us.

Then Virginia and Eric arrived. More talk. The talk stopped making sense to me. As I was getting Keith ready to go to sleep, I heard everyone in the kitchen talking and laughing and I wanted everyone gone. Wanted air. Wanted space, space to dissipate the fear and terror. Grief so extreme that it made me feel unable to move. And made me angry. I felt that Keith and I were in a different dimension from the rest of the world, and I didn't want to lose hold of where we were together. Voices making conversation, discussing everyday occurrences, grated on my nerves. I wanted all distractions gone. I wanted to get to know my fear. And I desperately wanted more time with Keith. Keith had said Tuesday—that was only four days away.

A panicky feeling that there wasn't enough time. Not enough time left; not enough time to be wasted on making conversation—even on saying good-bye and hello. And a kind of anger at the disparity between the discussions and the reality of Keith's death. What was everyone talking about? How can such words be spoken? It is both comforting and horrifying that the unspeakable can be spoken in the same breath as talks about the weather.

I went to bed nervous and upset. Afraid that maybe we were jumping to conclusions. Maybe there was life left to be lived for Keith. Hadn't we gone out just that morning? Keith in his wheelchair, Luke pushing him, I guiding with my hand, Robert along for security. Hadn't it been good? Couldn't there be more? Why were we pushing fate? Playing God?

Just a few nights ago Annie was here for the evening. She watched Luke while I did Keith's IV, then she cooked dinner. After dinner I was getting Luke ready for bed. I carried him into the kitchen to say good night to her while she was doing the dishes. Luke kissed her good night and said to me, "It's so cozy here."

This morning was a "nurse morning." Barbara, the weekend nurse came at eight. Victor at ten. A lab technician at ten-fifteen to take Keith's blood. Keith was a patient again. Bottles and tubes down the incinerator. Keith had diarrhea, a constant now. He had to go to the bathroom while he was on his DHPG IV. Barbara followed him to the bathroom, holding the IV bag, then instead of hooking it on the back of the bathroom door, she stayed with him while he was on the toilet. It made me furious. His privacy was invaded in his own home. On nurse mornings I see Keith as a helpless, frail man. It is wrong.

In the afternoon we saw Dr. Davis. Before our appointment I went to the drugstore and grocery store. Bought them out. Want to be well-stocked. Like being pregnant and waiting for the baby to come. Everything must be ready. Always.

Luke went off with Annie. At twelve-forty-five Keith and I left for Dr. Davis's office, with me pushing Keith in his wheelchair. I loved the feeling. We are a totally self-contained unit, my husband and I. I tuck my purse by his side and we take on the world. When I am pushing the wheelchair, I feel Keith's weight—I can bear that weight, protect him, because he is in my control. And we are powerful. Everything we see or confront is trivial, one-dimensional, irrelevant to us, except for the sun and the smells and the texture of the air. It didn't occur to me until we got home that I was happy doing what I had prayed would never happen—wheeling Keith in a wheelchair to see his doctor.

Dr. Davis seemed nervous about seeing us. Keith seemed nervous, too, but very determined. I am sure that Dr. Davis knew the nature of our visit because he ushered us into the examining room and then went and got a chair for me to sit in. Keith kept saying, "I need to talk to you," over and over. Dr. Davis kept saying, "Yes, I know." Keith said that he wanted to end his life. Dr. Davis stood silently looking at Keith for a few seconds, then he left the room and came back with a short paragraph, a living will saying that Keith, the undersigned, wanted to stop all life-support medication. I signed as the witness. Keith asked Dr. Davis how much time he had. Dr. Davis said he thought he'd have a few days before the virus would take over.

Dr. Davis helped Keith into the wheelchair. I could tell he was upset. It was a final good-bye. An unsaid good-bye. Dr. Davis didn't know what to say, but he was playing his part. He asked if I was warm enough. Did I have enough clothes on? We were a study in contrasts—Keith in his heavy sweater, down parka, knit cap; I in a light jacket. I pushed Keith outside onto the sidewalk and we hugged and cried. Tears of gratitude and relief on Keith's part, tears of amazement, appreciation, and love on mine. And pride. I was so proud of my husband. I was so proud of his courage. Keith's telling Dr. Davis that he wanted to die did not seem to come from desperation, it seemed to come from Keith's sense of right and wrong. He was doing the right thing. We felt our pride and dignity restored to us. I was so proud pushing Keith home.

The IV pole went out of the bedroom into the hallway. The medical supplies and medicines were trashed or closed up in boxes. After Annie came in with Luke we cleaned. I wanted things changed: fresh, new, and clean. Windows washed and the sticky medicine drips scrubbed off the floor. Airy and euphoric; teary and shaky. I want to make my way around the perimeter of our home, clean out the corners, stock the cupboards, celebrate all within it. And then bolt the doors. An unquenchable desire for privacy.

The pills Keith will need are hidden on the back of a high shelf in a vitamin jar. Keith took two of them that night to see what they were like. To get to know them.

March 29

Today was a quiet day, or as quiet as is possible with a two-year-old. Luke was home all day. Luke and Keith played together in bed, tickling each other and giggling. Each of us in our own way luxuriating the absence of the regime of medications. While Luke was napping I went into our bedroom to lie down with Keith. He asked me if I didn't want to practice my flute. I said I wanted to stay with him. He said, "Please, I like to hear you play." I went into the living room to play as I sometimes do, but this time I kept the doors between the bedroom and living room open.

March 30

This morning Keith said to me, "I feel better than I can remember. My body is thanking me."

Keith is already so much weaker than forty-eight hours ago. He no longer attempts to be moved into the living room to have lunch or see Luke. But his spiritual presence is stronger. I feel I have Keith back. His sense of humor has returned. He spent two hours gossiping and laughing with Virginia. He looks like himself to me now, not shadows of his relatives. (Sometimes in the past year I have woken up in the night, looked at Keith, and seen his father's face). I thought of England: I had seen Keith as an old, old man, past death. Now it seems as if he has gotten younger, back to his rightful present.

This afternoon while Luke was watching *Sesame Street* Virginia and I dissolved half of the pills in water and filled a syringe with the mixture. Then we wrapped it carefully and hid it. We wanted to have all the advance preparations out of the way— our minds must be clear for what is coming.

It is time for good-byes. Mine and Keith's I cannot comprehend, but there are other people involved. Part of me cannot stand for anyone other than Keith, Luke, and me to be in our home, but another part of me needs some social marking, some sharing of this event.

So I called my father, who had been wanting to visit Keith, and Dick. My father came this evening and sat by Keith lying in bed. When I saw my father out the door he said, "Keith seems at peace."

Then Dick came. It was his second visit to Keith here at home. I left Keith and Dick alone for a while, then went in to be with them. Dick said to Keith, "Luke doesn't ever have to know." That seemed wrong to me. I said, "I will never lie to my son." I am done with deceptions.

April 7

That was Monday evening. Tuesday morning a bouquet of wildflowers arrived from Dick with a note. It said: "It wasn't until I left that I could begin to put into thought what I felt being with you both. I never imagined such bravery, intelligence, and generosity could be—and in such depth and with such nobility of soul. You've taught me a lesson I never knew existed. I love you both and am with you."

The note helped calm me. An acknowledgment, a response to what we were doing, and the thought that it had touched someone else helped. It gave some strength. Virginia and I put the flowers on Keith's bedside table.

Tuesday was rainy and windy. Luke played at home. Our apartment was cozy. Sometimes when I walked into the bedroom I would find Keith smiling. Once I asked him why he was smiling. He said he was thinking about his life.

That morning Keith took a long bath and shower. He laughed and said he wasn't sure why he wanted to do that—who was going to see him?—but he felt it was important. I helped him cut his nails and shampoo his hair. It was like a ceremony, powdering his back and drying and combing his hair.

Part of my mind was doing a countdown: only fourteen hours left, only twelve hours left. The other part was saying that it didn't have to be tonight, it wouldn't be, it won't happen. We can have as many days as we want. This is good, this life is O.K. Maybe tomorrow the sun will be out and I can take Keith and Luke out. Luke can help me push Keith's wheelchair, or sit on Keith's lap and I can push them both. There are things we can look forward to. We can have another good day. Always a part of me repeating to myself, "He didn't say he was certain. Nothing is definite."

Pat, Larry, and Brandon came in the evening to take Luke out to dinner. I went into the bedroom to talk to Keith. He said that he felt strongly about tonight. I said that it was his decision. I went to cook dinner for us. Keith asked if he could watch me. He wanted to watch me in our home. He got out of bed and sat at the kitchen table. I desperately wanted to curl up in his lap and sob. But I couldn't. I couldn't let myself. I wouldn't be able to do what needed to be done if I got too close. I wouldn't be able to help him.

I had made a list of what I had to do in a notebook, hidden in the back of a kitchen drawer. I knew it by heart. The last instruction on the page was "Destroy this list."

Pat, Larry, and Brandon brought Luke home. Larry and I played with Brandon and Luke in the living room. Pat was saying goodnight to Keith in the bedroom. I heard her cry out and start to sob. I knew then that Keith was going to go through with it. He had said good-bye to her.

I got Luke ready for bed. Luke went into our bedroom and kissed Keith goodnight.

Then Keith and I got ready for bed. We set the alarm for 2 A.M. We didn't speak much, except to say that we both felt we were doing the right thing. There was a kind of relief. I curled up on Keith's shoulder. So peculiar: such a relaxed, deep sleep.

The alarm went off, miles away in my consciousness. I make some tea, look at my list. What am I doing? Are we packing for a trip? Go down the list. Check Luke. Get dressed. Keith and I smile at each other. I throw up; I cannot drink. I look at Keith. He looks into space. He looks determined. And he looks peaceful. So strong. So thin and so strong. Suddenly I know that I will get my strength from him. Suddenly I know that. I bring Keith what he needs.

His head propped up with pillows, Keith asks for the Bible. He lays our Bible on the bed and holds it in his left hand. His right hand reaches for me.

"You are my victory. Luke will be my triumph."

I stare into Keith's eyes. I look at my hand over his. He lies back on the pillows. His eyes close. I watch his chest go up and down. I breathe with him, for him. An eternity. Suddenly his eyes open, his back arches, he is looking past me. Staring, he smiles at something I cannot see. His breathing stops. I will sit here forever.

Then everything is cold—stiff and cold. I get up to open the curtains and let in the morning light.

When I think back to the days after Keith died what I remember is that the world seemed silent. A terrible silence because nothing rang true. For weeks after Keith died I thought about the sounds when Keith was sick. I mourned those sounds—Keith calling my name, the bath running, the IV control beeping when the medicine drip had stopped, Luke coming into our room in the morning and saying, "Hi, Daddy." After Keith died everything but the sound of Luke's voice was an interruption my pain could not tolerate, so I blocked everything else out.

Then one night I got out my journal. And its words rang true and strong. I wanted to hold its words, organize them—create with them something coherent and concrete that would help me remember, help me make sense of the unexplainable.

I am sure that everyone touched by tragedy wants—and needs to—tell their story. Tell it again and again. Try to make sense of it, try to fit it into the present. All those touched by tragedy must feel the frustration of not being able to find a place in the present for the events they hold in their hearts. I wanted to immortalize my loss. I wanted to find a place to put the anger I felt at the cruelty of life. These were the feelings that had prompted me to keep a journal in the first place. These were the feelings I had as I read and reread my journal through the night.

My journal helped me grieve my husband. But it did not help me resolve my anger. On the contrary. In the weeks after Keith's death my anger turned to rage. This was because I heard other stories. I received sympathy cards and sympathetic phone calls that said, "I know what you've been through. . . . I lost a lover [or a brother, a friend, a cousin]." I met a friend in the playground. She was shaking as she pushed her son on a swing. She said she had been to see an old friend of hers from college because she had heard he was sick. She had found him incoherent, emaciated and penniless, alone in his apartment, dying of AIDS without anyone to care for him. Keith's "buddy," now my friend, Wayne, called to say he had been diagnosed as having AIDS. He said he didn't know how to tell his parents because his brother also had AIDS, and he was afraid the news of his illness would destroy his mother.

Five months after Keith died, Luke started nursery school. A very fragile pair, Luke and I, entered a world where nobody knew about Luke's daddy. One morning, standing with the other parents watching our children play, one mother asked me what my husband had died of. I hesitated. Then I said, "He died of AIDS." She responded with silence.

As time went on other parents asked. Some I lied to, but mostly I told the truth. Most were very uncomfortable with the subject. Some were curious about the disease. But what struck me most was that all were ignorant about AIDS.

How can they not know? I thought. A tragedy beyond proportion is happening in your city—how can you not know? As my own grieving moved from numbness to pain I felt, as I reentered the world, that I was moving from a small sphere of society that was knowledgeable about AIDS to a world that was ignorant. And I became fearful for Luke.

I tell Luke about the man his father was. I tell him stories of his father's life—we dance to his father's music. But sometimes I am frightened that the father Luke constructs in his mind will not evolve from his memories and loving stories told by family and friends but rather be permanently clouded by the circumstances of his father's death. Will Luke have to confront this ignorance? This silence? What will it mean ten years from now to have a father who died from AIDS? As Luke's tears come and go through the years as he struggles to accept the death of his father, he is going to need help and support. What will he be told? What innuendos about AIDS has he already picked up?

I resolved to tell my story. The facts must be acknowledged. I began to feel that everyone touched by AIDS must tell his or her story until the stories are part of the fabric of our society. The stories can teach and enrich our lives so that we can respond to the horror of AIDS responsibly and with compassion. And, perhaps, not be as fearful of life's tragedies because we can face them openly, knowing our own power to shine in the face of darkness.

I put together this manuscript in an apartment of noise—the sounds of children playing. I appreciate the noise. I feel a terrible emptiness when I contemplate the irony that if Keith hadn't died I wouldn't appreciate what I now appreciate, enjoy what I now enjoy: the consolation prize of loss.

The present is made rich because of the past. And the past is made up of stories. We live in the present and approach the future endowed with our stories of the past. This story is part of my past. It is part of my son's legacy. As my son struggles to accept the death of his father, I pray this story will help him to understand what happened. Perhaps it will help others understand. May it help pave the way for my son's future.

GLOSSARY

AIDS (Acquired Immune Deficiency Syndrome): An acquired defect in a person's immune system that reduces the affected person's resistance to certain infections and cancers. AIDS is an acquired syndrome because it is a condition that cannot be transmitted by casual contact. It is generally believed to be caused by the Human Immunodeficiency Virus (HIV). To be classified as having AIDS a person must have developed one of the diseases specified by the Centers for Disease Control as an AIDS disease, such as Wasting Syndrome (Cachexia), Opportunistic Infections—such as Pneumocystis Carinii Pneumonia (PCP), Toxoplasmosis, Crytococcal Meningitis, or Cytomegalovirus (CMV)—cancers, such as Kaposi Sarcoma (KS) or lymphoma, or some neurological disorders.

AZT (Azidodeoxythimidine): Presently the only antiviral drug approved by the Federal Drug Administration for persons with

AIDS. AZT does not cure AIDS or prevent persons with AIDS (PWAs) from developing new infections. It does, however, reduce symptoms of HIV infection in those individuals who can tolerate its toxicity (estimated to be fifty percent of persons with AIDS). AZT causes anemia by suppressing the bone marrow.

CMV (Cytomegalovirus): A virus related to the herpes family. Severe CMV infections can cause colitis, hepatitis, pneumonia, and retinitis (an inflammation of the retina that can cause blindness).

KS Lesions: The manifestation of Karposis Sarcoma, a cancer of the capillaries that often occurs in persons with AIDS.

Opportunistic Infection: Any infection that would not necessarily be serious to anyone whose immune system is functioning properly but can cause serious illness or death in those individuals whose immune system is impaired.

PCP (Pneumocystis Carinii Pneumonia): A pneumonia caused by a common protozoal parasite that propogates rapidly in the lungs of persons with AIDS. It is the leading cause of death in AIDS.

TPN (Total Parenteral Nutrition): Intravenous nutritional feeding.

Tuberculosis: A species of bacteria called tuberculosis. Persons with AIDS are susceptible to MAI (Mycobacterium Avium Intracelluare), a species of tuberculosis that grows in the bone marrow.

Viral Encephalitis: Inflammation of the brain caused by a virus; not an uncommon cause of death for persons with AIDS.